THE ME I WANT TO BE

Simple Shifts To Authentic Wellbeing

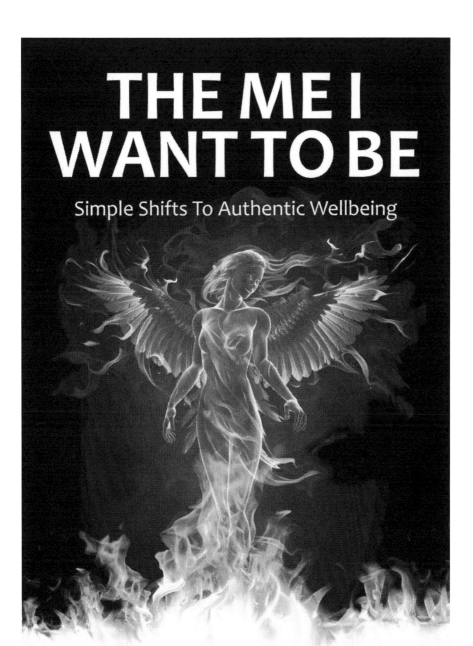

VICKI REBECCA

THE ME I WANT TO BE

Simple Shifts to Authentic Well-being

By Vicki Rebecca

Published by Vicreb Publishing
and also available at:
www.vickirebecca.com

Cover art and typesetting by:
Greenfield Design Associates Ltd
www.greenfielddesignassociates.co.uk

ISBN 9781533679598

About the Author

Vicki Rebecca's personal journey from glamour model to successful therapist both inspires and instructs. In *The Me I Want To Be*, Vicki shares the simple steps required to create an authentic and fulfilling life.

A UKCP accredited psychotherapist, trainer and supervisor; Vicki has an extensive background in health promotion, fitness training, yoga and meditation practice as well as professional qualifications to trainer level in psychotherapy, advanced clinical hypnosis and Neuro Linguistic Programming.

To find out more about Vicki: www.vickirebecca.com/about-me

Vicki wrote *The Me I Want To Be: Simple Shifts To Authentic Wellbeing* initially for the clients and students whom she has worked with for over twenty years. More especially she wrote it for those who could not manage to come along for sessions or classes because of cost or distance. It had always been a source of frustration to her that she could not help them too. So to make her work accessible to a larger audience she has written this book and recorded over ten hours of instruction and guided journeys to accompany it.

Those recordings are available from:
www.vickirebecca.com/resourcesandrecordings

I dedicate this book to my daughter,
for being her gorgeous, talented self
and the best reason ever to step up.

I love you.

Acknowledgments

I would like to thank my teachers.

Sue Washington, author, psychotherapist, friend, trainer and supervisor – my rock – without you, Sue, I would have never trawled through the academia of our profession – so glad I did.

Helen Belôt, Sekhem Grand Master. I sat at Helen's feet for a week in Australia drinking her wisdom and energy. During a fiery exchange, Helen reflected to me some of life's hardest lessons, forced me to look within. I did. She also told me when I forgave the one who hurt me most I would have truly arrived. That day has come – thank you.

So many other wonderful teachers: Egyptian Sekhem with Simon Treselyan, NLP with Richard Bandler; Meditation, Mindfulness and Yoga with Daizan Skinner. Also Jonathan Cohen, Sue Richter, Trish Troup, Paddy O'Ryan... the list goes on.

My biggest teachers have been the groups that sat with me as I taught, my clients, and the women with whom I meditated as we worked through our daily stress and life's ups and downs.

I thank my mother for always encouraging me, and my father for being the wisest being on the planet. My friends for being inspirational and amazing, and a special thanks to those who listened to me rant for the entire period of my divorce – no amount of psychology can ever replace that! To the wonderful woofers (the young people who have worked in our home in exchange for bread, board and learning our Scottish ways) who took over the daily do thus facilitating the finishing of this book.

My grandma, for teaching me the basics of herbs from her garden, the qualities of her soups and other foods, how to dowse for the sex of an unborn child and dream of the face of your husband to be. The younger adults in the family called it her 'old wives tales.' My grandma was with us until she was ninety-six and was a great, great grandma. She was my first teacher.

I would also like to thank Ros Greenfield at Greenfield Design Associates who pushed me through the final polishing.

Special thanks to my loyal girls, Cat, Jill, Josie and Ewa. Jacqui Scott for the love, patience and friendship she brought to the audio production - without those qualities I would have never managed the recordings that are such an integral part of this work. John Harten, who helped unscramble my words, made me look forward to feedback and turned this writer into an author.

My deepest thanks - I love you all.

Preface

Celtic Warrior Woman
by Simon Treselyan

The sun cascaded its rays and warmed the sands as it had done for millennia before the first Egyptian laid claim to the land. The smiles of those having landed in Cairo reflected the warmth and the shine of wonder. I had seen the look many times in different forms in differing classes. Seekers of truth and initiates of an energy rightly called 'The Power of Powers' - Egyptian Sekhem.

Her hair was like that of a lion's mane; her compact and fit stature indicated a discipline to her art of yoga. She looked like she meant business. Her name was Vicki Rebecca and she had entered the land of the Pharaohs, perhaps not for the first, or last, time. Our next couple of weeks in sacred sites and ritual were to enhance and cement a friendship that would last through the sands of time.

There is nothing more powerful it is said than an Idea whose time has come…Women have been, will be and are Warriors! As we know the Celtic spirit is fierce and uncompromising in attack and warming and compassionate in peace. When co-joined with the purity of her spirit and the power of her teaching you have here, a unique Celtic Warrior Woman in Vicki. I am delighted and honoured to be involved in Vicki's work, as a testament to her continued path to the Mastery I believe began on the shores of the Nile.

With the world as it is, it is imperative that Women now stand up and create a new future. 'But Warriors?' you may ask … History acknowledges what we know to be true. Anyone who doesn't believe in the Warrior power of the Woman needs only to try and come between her and her children and they will find out rather quickly how this power can be unleashed.

The power of the Warrior is distinctly feminine in form and Vicki represents this energetic and values based aspect. 'Warriors' are different from normal people. They have always been the Custodians of the tribe and represent all that is good about the culture they serve. Warriors protect and defend; they will fight for those that are unable to protect themselves. In the past Women have always been the natural protectors of children and the home without which the men would have no future. It did not take long for women to realise that if their soldier men were defeated that they could expect no mercy from an invading force. They became Warriors by default, certainly not lacking courage to do what sometimes has to be done.

Women now are truly finding their power and it will be the unity of opposites that will determine the success of our species. Vicki is a prime example of this and it is reflected in her teachings. She is unique in that she has what can be perceived as having a male strength and focus, aligned with her obvious female compassion and awareness, we have the co-joining forces of success just as God designed it to be. A Woman in her Power, without fear and absolutely clear that her position is earned.

Like anything of value in life there is a cost to achieve success. You will, spend hours reading this book and taking valuable time doing the exercises. Some of these may be challenging, for you can never solve the problem with the same mind-set that created it in the first place. This is not theoretical, sugar-coated rhetoric; this is tried and tested, proven material that is aptly demonstrated in Vicki's life. If you are prepared to take the time and effort you will be rewarded with a similarly vibrant life. In this Vicki is an excellent guide and coach.

Do you have what to takes to demand of this life the Power of the Warrior for your own? If you had the choice would you wish to be the Victor or the Victim? For in that you will always have a choice. In Vicki's expansive and ground-breaking book, The Me I Want To Be, there now exists the recipes and call to action for women everywhere to be self-determined by right, not luck or allowance.

Never before in history has there been so much need for the Warrior Woman in this world and it corresponds with the opportunities the modern

World has for Fearless Women that are standing up and making a difference. A difference many of your Sisters never experienced.

Be that difference today and ensure all of our futures tomorrow.

Simon Treselyan spent 19 years in Military Special Forces and is a well known figure in the Personal and Human Development field. His Books 'Who Dares for Success' and 'Courage Conquers All Things' are now joined by 'The Order of the Nephilim,' which is about to be made into a major Hollywood film.

www.starfirebooks.com

Vicki Rebecca

Foreword

I can only smile when I think of the all adventures this book has brought to me, yet a year before publication I realised I wasn't ready to fully step into the ownership of all it contained.

Authenticity!

The chapters, which are the fruits of my daily labour were easy. Helping others master body, mind, emotions, past and destiny is my 9-5. However, when I got down to the nitty gritty and asked myself the questions: What IS it that I really want to share? What is it that others will want to hear that will truly help them change their lives and be who they really want to be?

I had to have a big think.

In the end I realised I had a story about finding and expressing my own authenticity, my own voice, my core and my strength. I wanted to share my discovery of something within that made me realise I was worth saving. There had been a time when I felt so small, so wrong, and so dirty deep inside that I convinced myself I had been dealt a joker card. I played over and over in my mind this awful 'realisation' that there was 'something' completely wrong with me. It was a nonspecific sneaky slippery defect that eluded definition and therefore cure and which showed up in various guises all my life. I possessed a golden outward appearance, and a keen enough intellect, yet I would always malfunction.

There are still times when I plummet into the despair of self-doubt, when I feel the shame and ask myself "How dare I?" The difference is now, at long last, I have a method of being still and solid inside. I have the resources to find peace of mind, comfort in my own skin and the connection to all things in this truly amazing universe.

Nothing has honed it more than the writing of this book.
In the end, this book has enabled me to take the final step out of self-

judgment and into the fire of my own transformation. This is what I am living and loving right now. What I offer was gathered during the journey away from life as a glamour girl and heroin addict, to who I am now. I love the person I am now. That transition took me through the steps I share with you: mastering the body, mind, past, eventually the emotions too, and including the metaphysical development, which for me centred in ancient Egypt.

So, *The Me I Want To Be* is a joint effort of my own personal-development: all types of fitness, meditation yoga and energy work. What I have found to work in my professional practice: hypnotherapy and psychotherapy; and what I discovered through esoteric study that the ancients took as their way of life. These are the steps that led me from addiction to the glowing health and happiness I enjoy today. I now hold deeply as a truth the knowing that from every challenge and every place where I thought I was undone, something better came out of it. I have seen the same in my clients. I share here the practices that really made the difference, and a little more of my journey.

During that final 'thinking' time, pre-publication, the overwhelming message from friends and clients who'd read the book, was to be myself. I received lots of comments like: "I've read all that stuff before, but the way you put it, I totally get it."

So here I am, yes, I've done 'all of that stuff,' and its energy permeates these pages, the recordings, classes and retreats. But I write as I teach and help: straight, simple, and from the heart.

I hope you like it.

Vicki Rebecca

You are more than you know you are.
And you already know all you need to know...

Contents

Preface   Celtic Warrior Woman by Simon Treselyan

Chapter 1   Self Mastery 1

Chapter 2   Mastering the Body 13

Chapter 3   Mastering the Mind 31

Chapter 4   Mastering the Emotions 43

Chapter 5   Mastering the Past 57

Chapter 6   Mastering Destiny 73

Chapter 7   Living the Mystery 93

Glossary 105

Afterword 109

Vicki Rebecca

Chapter 1

SELF MASTERY

The ancients mastered their physical and their metaphysical bodies. They mastered their thoughts, emotions, energy; even their soul's transit to the afterlife; and naturally, their beloved Egypt, which they believed was heaven on Earth.

You too can achieve new levels of mastery beginning with self-knowledge.

I fell in love with Egypt the moment I set foot on her soil, and as clichéd as it sounds, it felt like coming home.

Ancient Egypt gave the rest of the world a vast amount of its knowledge and there is still so much we can learn. The ancient Egyptians were master architects, applying the knowledge of sacred geometry like the phi ratio to building the pyramids. They were master stonemasons, astrologers and astronomers. They studied law, including the universal laws. They studied alchemy and chemistry of all types, including medicine, working with perfumes and oils, creating the elixirs and essences used for anointing and other rituals. They studied physical science, mastering their bodies through yoga, and they were keen practitioners of Tantra. You can see the pride they took in their appearance from the perfect physiques painted on the temple walls. They left us depictions of surgical operations including cosmetic surgery and engravings of massage and of childbirth; no part of life was omitted from the temple art.

They had a thorough understanding of the interaction of mind, body, spirit and all the implications thereof. They mastered their thoughts and emotions through meditation and other spiritual practices. In the mystery schools, after experiencing each emotion and sitting with it, they'd learn to flit from emotion to emotion, to summon each emotion at will and use it as a platform to the spiritual realms. Priests were the official sorcerers working their magic in all areas of life, including against the enemies of Egypt. They learned the mysteries through years of training and finally underwent an initiation in the King's Chamber that would actually imprint the mysteries onto their energy bodies.

There were no certificates saying 'master' dished out for simply attending a one-day seminar in those days. They entered the mystery schools at seven years of age and they served and served, and they practiced, and practiced. Then they had to prove themselves by demonstrating the skills taught. If you've ever seen pictures of them with their lions, you'll see there were no chains: the master would control the lion with the power of his mind alone, and of course the price of failure in the King's Chamber was certain death. This was the real thing, that's for sure. The ancients must have known and faced their fears in many ways.

I was impressed. To become a master at anything takes ten thousand hours and surely must take a level of self-knowledge deeper than most of us ever achieve. That's something to aspire to. I don't mean to say your dream is to undergo a three-day rite in a smelly sarcophagus or to tame a lion, but wouldn't it be great to borrow some of their wisdom and practices to achieve a contentment-filled quality life that REALLY suits you?

That's what we are going to do.

We'll do it by embracing change from the inside out. In the end, there is only one thing that has to be developed: and that is the self. The true essence of the self needs to be developed in order to claim the fullness of the future we desire, not just for one of us, but for all of us. We'll do that through self-study and practice. You are more, you can change and the shifts are smaller than you think! I'll guide you through it.

However, before we get into it I'd like to say a little about the practicalities. I recognise we're all coming to this from slightly different backgrounds and you may well already know some of the steps within. So the idea is that you read the book, then go through the Resources and Recordings (available on www.vickirebecca.com/resourcesandrecordings) following the exercises and listening to the recordings, filling in any gaps in your current skill set. For instance, the mastery chapters begin with mastering the body, as that was how it came to me. My body was already strong despite the abuse I'd given it, so I began from my strength. It was encouraging. However, when it comes to working through the resources, feel free to do it in an entirely different order if that's what suits you.

First let's look at relaxation, as it doesn't matter how enlightened you are; in today's world we can all do with a little more relaxation. Then we'll delve into self-knowledge, because to develop personally and spiritually you first need to know yourself and your own truth. We'll establish a connection with that truth which will take us out of illusion and help us remember that we already have it all within.

LEARN TO RELAX

First you need to relax enough to hear the messages sent to you from the self in the centre of your being as opposed to the ranting, frazzled self that deafens you to your soul's truth. It is your soul's truth that will empower you through the struggles life inevitably brings.

Two Perfect Systems

You are an amazing being and Mother Nature has provided for you well: she's given you Two Perfect Systems.

Once upon a time, way back in the Stone Age when humanity was in its infancy, we developed a survival tool – a hormonal and chemical spending spree if you like – called the fight-or-flight response. The fight-or-flight response evolved so that when the larder was bare and bellies were empty, and Fred, our friendly caveman, had no other choice but to get the spear out, he had the faculty to summon that extra drive needed to make the kill. This faculty operated so that as he and the rest of the hunters drew near the hunting ground, they started feeling revved up: the brain telling the body to release chemicals priming the hunters for fighting or fleeing, so that by the time they had the animal in their sights, they would be fully focused and ready to make the kill. That effort, then the dragging of the beast home, would use up the discharged chemicals so that complete recovery came naturally after the inevitable celebration shindig and rest to follow.

It's as simple as that: a perfect system, the stress response.

Our biology still provides for such emergencies, although these days we rarely encounter a dangerous beast on the warpath. These days our stressors are quite different to Fred's (and Wilma's, who stoically endured the pre-hunt revving-up ceremony and post-hunt boasting!). Nowadays, instead of a large, toothy beast, we have a difficult boss. We have no need to go out hunting, but most of us feel we have to show up for work five or six days a week. We rarely feel hunger in our bellies, but we do spend hours ingesting radio waves from telephones; suffering badly-programmed cyber assistants from call centres; waiting in traffic jams and choking down plastic food. Unfortunately, these days, spear throwing just isn't on the agenda; that kind of physical action went out with clubbing Wilma on the head. However, we find our stress response activated in situations where, as much as we'd love to, there's just no opportunity to discharge those chemicals and hormones without the possibility of ending up in jail.

So lacking an appropriate means of discharge, stress takes its toll on the body and mind, not to mention the soul. With the complications of our modern society, stress may continue indefinitely, which is very damaging and can end up compromising the whole system, leading to dis-ease in every way. But do not fear: clever Mother Nature also gave us the antidote. Just as we have the stress response as one of the body's built-in systems, so there is the innate relaxation response, programmed to come to the rescue by undoing the effects of stress: another perfect system, a system that is REALLY good for you.

There is, however, a slight difference: a loud bang would probably startle you and get the stress reaction going through your body, and the sight of a sabre-toothed tiger in the back garden would have you up the nearest tree in a nanosecond. Why, I've even seen my mother jump on top of the coffee table that fast at the sight of a field mouse, and that was when she was eighty-two!

However, what if I said: "One, two, three – you're under"?

Well, maybe eventually you could train yourself to relax and go into a trance when prompted in that way, but generally it just wouldn't happen. The relaxation response needs to be purposefully sought and practiced. There are times when the relaxation response does occur naturally, for instance when you sit on the beach watching the ocean, but let's face it – how often does that happen?

So unlike its stressful counterpart, the relaxation response is not automatic; you must deliberately put time aside for it and practice! In other words, you need to learn to relax. It's really quite simple: find the time and space, somewhere comfortable where you will not be disturbed, find a method that suits you and then practice, practice, practice! Don't worry, just relax and let me guide you. Honest, it's that simple.

The thing is, you cannot even begin to know yourself properly and thus uncover the powerful resources you already possess without taking the time to relax and find them for yourself. So if you haven't already done so, this is a good moment to enjoy our first journey together, introduction to relaxation.

Preparation, Practice and the Stairway of Learning

Whatever happens, don't worry about it. Maintain a passive attitude and let relaxation come at its own pace; with practice, the relaxation response will come. Sometimes it takes several practice sessions to become aware of the effects. Keep going; practice is the key. Relaxation is a skill, and like any skill, the more you practice, the better you will get at it. Without practice, you will not improve. To benefit, you must actually do it. Repetition works, so practice, practice, practice!

I see a huge difference in results between clients who show up every week for their hypnosis session and those who show up plus practice daily at home. Just think of the difference in results you'd get if you went to the gym every day as opposed to once a week. It's obvious, isn't it? Who would ever be able to play chopsticks, far less Beethoven's 9th, without practice? Imagine hoping to win a horse-jumping contest or tennis game after only one coaching session.

Language habits take twenty-one days of regular practice before they become 'unconscious.' We know it takes the same amount of practice to reprogram new thinking habits, new emotional habits, and new behavioural habits. But listen to this: there are seventeen sets of three-week periods in a year, so if you practice one new, key habit for twenty-one days, in a year's time you will have transformed your life!

Each time you do something, your brain lays down a neural pathway, and each time you repeat that thing, these neural connectors fire off. The more they fire together, the more they wire together. So practice doesn't make behaviour perfect – it makes it unconscious. Once these life-improving habits become automatic through practice, guess what: the quality of your life improves.

To encourage themselves, students in our relaxation class resolve to practice every day for a hundred days, ticking each one off on the calendar so they can see their progression. When I learn something new, I like to remind myself of the stairway of learning. It goes like this: at first you don't even know that you don't know something. For example, you don't know there is something called the relaxation response that can improve your life; you are unconsciously unskilled. Then someone tells you that there is something that you don't know about, so you become uncomfortable, being conscious now that you are unskilled in that area. So you read a book or go to a class and learn the basics. You are still uncomfortable, though; you've been told what to do but are not really confident that you are doing it right. If you keep practicing until eventually it becomes automatic, you will become unconsciously skilled: you won't even think about it anymore, and you'll have reached the top of the stairway!

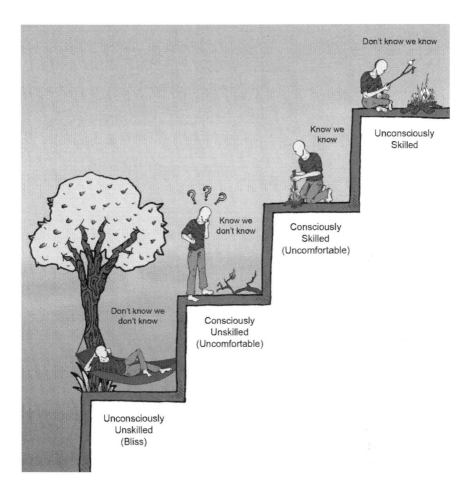

Repetition is the mother of all skill!

The relaxation response and other techniques that are included in the resources for this book have been truly tried and tested by me, my students, my clients, and my friends. They are the key to opening doors and changing your life. The benefits are outstanding. As a therapist and trainer, I see people every day who turn their lives around purely through learning how to relax. At the classes, the most common feedback I hear the following week is "I slept like a log." Learning to relax is the basis of all the tools you will learn. So be gentle, kind and patient with yourself as you learn new ways of thinking and being. Treat yourself as you would someone you really loved. If you don't believe me, that's OK. Just give me twenty-one days!

Everything good that you wish for those around you, you deserve for yourself, so give that to yourself and GLOW with inner confidence!

DEVELOP YOUR SELF ESTEEM

Just by checking out your response to relaxation, already you know a little more about you, correct? I know it is; you see, your response, whatever it was, is information about you! Once you get relaxed enough, your self-awareness will develop and you will more easily hear yourself, get to know your inner voice, responses and behaviours. Whatever that is, you can acknowledge it and then simply let it pass, for example:

"I am a fidgeting, ranting fruit and nut case."

Acknowledge it and continue to practice. That's all. At the same time begin to be kinder to yourself to build up self-esteem. You certainly need it if you call yourself names like that! Self-esteem is the quality above all others that determines how you respond to the circumstances in your life. Just as stress debilitates your life, so a robust self-esteem improves it. Lack of it may be why you picked up this book in the first place.

You may be a confident individual, but confidence and self-esteem are not necessarily the same thing. Some of us can make a great presentation at work, pass through school top of our year, have all the outer wrappings of success, but nevertheless have self-esteem issues. Perhaps you struggle with both aspects. It doesn't matter what stage you are at; you can learn to look after yourself a little bit more.

Begin to address those issues now. Develop your self-esteem by really paying yourself some attention. When I ask clients what they like to do just for themselves, often they just don't know. Do you know? Do you know what you like doing just for you, and when you last did it, and have you wondered if you could do it more often? What else could you do for yourself? What can you do for yourself right now? Write it down, accept it as truth, and then give it to yourself. I mean it! I have seen so many clients become magically more assertive and begin to tackle all sorts of other problems when they begin to give to themselves. This is how you get your needs met, guaranteed.

Separate Needs and Wants

You may need to separate your needs from your wants. Sometimes you think you need a holiday, but if you break it down, you might want a holiday or would like a holiday, but often what you really need is just a break, just some time out.

The solution can be in the little things like a pampering bath with your favourite oils, a cuppa with your feet up or a short walk. If I take Ted (my chocolate lab), out for longer than the usual twenty minutes that can be enough. Even the twenty minutes can allow that shift in gear. A break can be even shorter than that: a stretch out on the carpet, floor or chair. I teach a four-minute relaxation for stress, and clients are always delighted by how much better they feel even after such a short time.

Little things like playing your favourite piece of music will do. Having Sunday morning in bed with the papers; cooking yourself a special meal and sitting at the table to eat it. Surrounding yourself with candlelight. Do these little things often, and then you can build up to more.

Take twenty-four, even twelve hours out, get in your car and drive, check into a bed-and-breakfast, do nothing but enjoy the bath and someone else cooking the breakfast. I've done that and returned feeling like I'd had a week off. The main thing is that it's something for YOU!

You don't really need to go into the city and scorch the plastic; you can drive to that special little shop and buy the most beautiful crystal or handmade soap for a few pennies. Enjoy a cuppa in a special coffee shop pretending for a moment you have all the time in the world. If you remember to differentiate between needs and wants, that trip around the world could become a five-year long-term plan or a night away next month. A month on a desert island may actually mean that you simply need a few hours' extra sleep, a hug and some sunshine. An hour-long cry may actually be finished in less than ten minutes if you only let yourself have it.

If you struggled to think of what it is that you like, it may simply be that it's just been too long. Perhaps you need to ask what you would like if you did know what that was. It could also be that you are spending too much time trying to meet someone else's needs in the hope that your needs will be met after theirs. It doesn't work like that. You have to put your focus on you, make yourself the priority. No one is an endless reservoir of energy. We all need to get something back. In other words, if your battery is too low, how can you even think about giving your neighbour a jump-start? If you keep putting your needs off, the consequences will be enormous. Self-neglect leads to bitterness, resentment, anger and ill health, and then you'll have a whole different set of needs to attend to!

The more you can look after yourself, the better and the happier you feel and the more energy you will have to get on with life.

Looking Within - embrace change from the inside out

To ensure you are meeting your needs, you need to know what they are. So to begin your journey of self-mastery, you need to learn to know yourself. I mean being honest. Not the "I am such a terrible person" type of honesty, although we can all have times where we say, "I'll do that differently next time," or, "I really ought to make amends here," but berating yourself really doesn't help. I don't mean that you have to "big yourself up" either. I am not talking about self-knowledge from ego, but self-knowledge from the soul. A knowledge that will help you see the gifts already within and realise that hiding and avoiding your shame and tears just leads to more shame, more tears, and other escalating issues. So together let's take a further step into self-knowledge with Temple of the Heart: Looking Within – if you wish, you can listen right now. The reference is at the end of Develop Your Self-Esteem in the Resources and Recordings. It is a tool to use many, many times every day to establish the connection and keep it strong. The more you do it, the more your heart will speak directly to you. When you give yourself the small answers many times every single day, the big answers tend to sort themselves out.

We spend far too much time anal-ysing. I remember my Dad saying, "Up here for thinking (head) and down there for dancing (feet)," and it is true, but he should have also pointed to his chest and said in here for knowing. The brain is great for working out the budget, but for the deeper questions, to know your truth you must enter the heart.

Find your truth in the wisdom of your heart and give yourself what you need right now!

Take the simple steps of relaxing, listening to your heart, and giving yourself what you need to look after yourself continuously and you will reap rich rewards. You are ready to begin. In keeping with the ancient Egyptian approach, let's do it with intent.

Intent

The first step to self-mastery is intent, so plant the seed right now: it is time to make your statement of mastery – your first initiation.

Ask yourself what you intend to receive from this journey. What is it you really want? If you are not sure, you may want to look at what kinds of things have been coming up as you look into your heart moment to moment. You may want to ask yourself what you love, what you hate, what you are passionate about, and what drives you. Are you living the life of your dreams? If you're not sure, let me put it another way: Do you want things to stay the way they are right now? If they did, where would you be six months from now, a year from now, five, even ten years from now? Scary? So ask again, what is it that you REALLY want? Then ask yourself why. Why is it you want that, what will you gain from it, and will it feel good when you have it?

When you get really clear about how you want to feel, you'll do what it takes. So let yourself feel it, see it happening right now, step into it, and let your imagination play around with it. Let yourself feel passionate and fired up, and realise how fantastic you'll feel when you get it. Once you hit the spot, you'll know. You'll be dreaming your desire and letting that vision pull you forward through the next steps. If you can dream it you can live it, I'll show you how.

Choose what you REALLY want, then watch as the universe guides you to master your destiny.

First write your statement of mastery. A short paragraph will do, something like this: "I, Vicki, intend to live my life in joy, love and laughter as I realise how to live the greatest and grandest expression of my being and help others do the same."

Then ask: Is that the future you are now committed to? Are you ready to embrace the changes it will bring, changes that will occur from the inside out?

If so, start immediately taking action in that direction. Be honest with yourself, and keep checking – is this going to get me to my goal? If so, keep on doing it! If not, ask what else you need to do, how else you need to be, shift a little in one direction or another, especially in your attitude to yourself. Tiny adjustments make the difference between doing OK and being an amazing being living an incredible life. You won't be as far out as you think; the secret to success is usually very simple.

"Don't worry about what the world needs. Ask what makes you come alive and do that, because what the world needs is people who have come alive." Howard Thurman

Now that you're learning to relax, have established the practice of self-knowledge and began building self-esteem, you'll feel good enough to embrace the next lessons. These are the lessons of mastery, the foundation to the life you aspire to, just as they were in the ancient mystery schools.

Let's start with the physical body.

Chapter 2

MASTERING THE BODY

The ancient Egyptians took pride in the perfect physique.

You too can cherish the temple you live in.

You are not this physical body...
You borrow it while you walk this beautiful Earth.

It is true you are not your body, but the body is where you live, so it is best not to wait until you are ready to drop it before giving it the honour and respect it deserves. If you think of your body as belonging to someone else – would you really treat it as badly as you sometimes do?

We die in three minutes without oxygen, and in days without water, yet so few of us practice breathing techniques or hydrate ourselves properly. Few of us learn what kind of fuel our bodies need for optimum energy and vitality, what kind of exercise can make us come alive, nor realise that it is ourselves that manages our physiological state and the ensuing combination of chemicals that lets us exude glowing good health. Perhaps it is time for a rethink.

Take Care of your Body: cherish and revere the temple you live in

• Learn to breathe

• Cultivate the hydration habit

• Learn about nutrition

• Learn to move yourself and keep moving

• Learn to master your physiological state

Before you know it, you will be fitter and stronger, your energy will improve, and you will begin to experience the inner glow of deep self-acceptance

Breathe

If we die within minutes without oxygen, it can be no surprise that a common cause of illness is improper breathing. Learning to breathe properly has such a profound effect that it is a joy to help those with anxiety-based conditions and see their delight at how much better they feel in just a matter of seconds. They can be a touch cynical when I mention abdominal breathing; maybe they have tried it before without effect, or it just seems too easy. However, with guidance, they find the relaxation response and feel their anxiety gone or massively reduced for the first time in weeks, months or even years. So simple. Why do we overlook the obvious so often?
Take time to practice the art of breathing. You breathe all the time: you may as well learn to do it in a way that benefits you the most.

Water

"You are not just what you eat; you are what you drink."
Dr Batmanghelidj

Water is the elixir of life, yet few of us drink enough of it. We can live for weeks and weeks without food, but only around a week without water. Water is the basis of all life and that includes your body: your muscles are 75 percent water; your blood, the body's transportation system for nutrients, 82 percent water; your lungs, providing your body with oxygen, 90 percent water; your brain, control centre of your body, is 76 percent water; even your bones are 25 percent water. You are mostly water. Your planet is mostly water. You must drink. Dehydration can be disastrous. Water is crucial to your wellbeing.

A dry mouth is one of the last signs of being dehydrated!

Side effects of chronic dehydration are stress, backache, weight gain, allergies, blood pressure and Alzheimer's; is that what you're after? When you are thirsty, you're already dehydrated. Your urine should run clear; if it's yellow, be concerned, and if it's dark, you're severely dehydrated! Every day you ought to be drinking half of your body weight (in pounds) in ounces of water, approximately 2 -3 litres depending on your size, the climate and the exercise you do.

Dr Batmanghelidj, who is an expert on hydration, escaped execution after the Iranian revolution by serving as a doctor in prison. During this time, when medication was not available, he discovered the medicinal value of water. He went on to make the study of water and vitality his life's work. Batmanghelidj concluded that water plays an important role not only in maintaining health, but also in curing disease. While modern medicine has labelled various states of dehydration as disease, Dr Batmanghelidj's work on Unintentional Chronic Dehydration (UCD) shows it contributes to, and even produces, pain and many degenerative diseases that could be prevented and treated simply by increasing water intake on a regular basis.

"You're not sick; you're thirsty. Don't treat thirst with medication."
Dr Batmanghelidj

The quality of the water you drink is also important, and I don't just mean where it comes from. Emoto Masaru, the Japanese entrepreneur and author of Messages from Water, claims that human consciousness has an effect on the molecular structure of water. Emoto's hypothesis, evolved over the years of his research, is that high-quality water forms beautiful and intricate crystals, while low-quality water has difficulty forming crystals. He claims that positive changes to water crystals can be achieved through prayer, music, or by attaching written 'words of intent' to a container of water. His photographs show the visual difference between the effects of the good vibes and the bad vibes on the crystals. Amazing!

So, if water holds intent, and since you are three-quarters-plus water, it means that every day you can choose your state with the simple act of drinking pure, clear water set aside for yourself. Honour it in a favourite jug or container, hold it with love and infuse it with intent. Why not? It's body-mind wisdom at its best. The ancient Egyptians, who well understood the influence of the mind upon the body, would write a spell on a piece of parchment in water-soluble ink then place it in water. The 'patient' would drink the magic of the words, so why not drink the magic of your own words of intent?

Drink with love and make each sip filled with intention.

Exactly the same applies to what you eat, your fuel.

Food

You've heard the old adage "you are what you eat," but have you ever stopped to think exactly how true that is? Healthy and nutritious foods boost how you feel in general and give you that healthy glow. They help you perform at your best in every aspect of your life; give you energy as opposed to stealing it; help process your emotions; prevent and fight disease; restore, rejuvenate and regenerate you. That is because food is not just energy.

Food is medicine, food is fuel

During my early thirties, I was suffering some kind of rheumy condition; my joints were swelling up, especially one knee. I would get out of bed like an old granny, hardly able to straighten my leg. My diet was awful, I had gained weight, and I was depressed. Both of my parents have arthritis, but my mother, unlike most of her generation, is a great believer in natural remedies and told me about a book on diet and arthritis. I tried it.

I embarked on a one-month elimination diet during which I ate fish (mostly salmon), sweet potatoes, carrots, pears and kiwis; I think that was it. Slowly, other foods were re-introduced one at a time. I will never forget the day I had to re-introduce cheese. I was quite far down the line of knowing what suited me and what didn't by that time and there had been no great surprises until then. I had to eat a decent-sized chunk of cheese and did so before I left home for the day. By the time I got 10-15 minutes along the road, I was in tears. I started thinking about someone I wasn't getting along with, then played out an imaginary conversation in my head with them (one I was unlikely to ever have), the result of which was so frustrating I ended up crying. I couldn't believe what was going on for me – the cheese! I would have never believed it if I hadn't experienced it myself; no wonder they say it gives you nightmares.

Do I live without cheese? No, thankfully that hasn't been necessary. As I said, my diet had been awful. We can get a build-up of things, which may well be fine in moderation but fatal if we've overdone them for years. So yes, I kept it out of my diet for a while and then reintroduced it slowly. I love parmesan to accompany my occasional pasta dish and a lump of good-quality cheddar now and again, but never again would I overindulge in that particular product.

So I know first-hand just how much food can affect us. I'm certainly not the only one. A good friend, Kerrie, was in so much pain she could barely walk until she started eating eighty percent raw – miraculously she became pain free. Another friend, Hilary, recovered from debilitating ME through a similar diet. Do you know what's good for you, in general and specifically?

I bet you could more easily name your favourite wine, coffee, or restaurant rather than what nutrients to ingest. Think about what you allow yourself to take into your body. Sugar – masses of it everywhere, and the only nutritional value it has is the instant energy hit it gives. High fructose corn syrup is even worse so please don't be deluded by the "alternatives."

What Is Good For You?

The UK government put out guidelines in the 1980s that we ought to eat less and exercise more, and apparently we do – so how come the rate of obesity is higher than ever? It can only be what we are putting into ourselves. The food industry is far from innocent: read your labels, and think about it before you eat it. Here's what my friend said about it:

"Eat less and do more. A simple case of calories in, versus calories out. Ironically, we have been exercising more and eating less, but also getting fatter, especially since the 1980s. This was when the low-fat mantra really took a grip. Weight for weight, fat provides more calories compared with carbohydrates or protein. However, once these are swallowed, each nutrient is metabolised differently; all calories are not the same! Nevertheless, the food manufacturing industry created a vast range of low-fat foods. We kept buying these foods, we kept eating them ... but did not lose weight. This is because by taking out the fat, something needs to be replaced. That something is usually sugar or refined starches – which behave like sugar in the body. These are cheap fillers, which bulk out food, replace the fat ... but make us fat.

So it is the sugars, starches and refined carbohydrates that make us fat. These cause the hormone insulin in the body to rise. High insulin levels signal to the body to convert sugar into fat – and store this fat for a future need. However, this future never comes as if the next snack or meal is full of sugar or cheap fillers, insulin remains high and we keep piling on fat. A more effective way to lose fat is to replace cheap processed food with real foods – fatty fish, eggs, whole milk, mature cheese, grass-fed beef, free-range chicken and your favourite vegetables glazed with organic butter or a homemade cheese sauce. Low-calorie and low-fat diets don't work in the long term. Eat real food, lose weight, gain health ... and stay that way." Dr Chris Fenn

Ask someone who was around before World War II whether there was such a problem with weight back then and what they ate. There would have been less variety of fruit (fewer imports but also fewer pesticides), so they would have eaten what fruit they could grow and local vegetables in season, fish if they lived near the sea, and meat from the butcher if they could afford it. Sounds good, doesn't it? And there's more:

Eat 70 percent water-based foods, of which 80 percent is veg and 20 percent fruit; 10 percent veg and fish proteins; 10 percent complex carbs; plus 10 percent oils.

If your body is over 75 percent water, it makes sense to eat at least 70 percent water-based or plant-based foods – fruit, veg, and salad – as this allows your body to cleanse itself. Let's face it: if you are not cleansing your body, you are clogging it up. So to gain maximum nutrients, eat as much raw foods as you can: uncooked, or cooked below a certain temperature, unprocessed, organic and wild! Include nuts, seeds, or sprouted whole grains. Raw may also include unpasteurized fermented foods such as sauerkraut, kefir, or kombucha. Raw foods can be life-changing. There's lots of choice – almonds, carrots, dates, avocados, limes, celery, cauliflower...

The rest ought to be 10 percent carbohydrates, 10 percent protein and 10 percent oils. Yes, the body also needs fats – healthy, healing, essential fatty acids Omega 3 and Omega 6 to function; without them, the cells start to break down. You also need to maintain a proper balance between acid and alkaline food. Too much acidity causes the body to produce insulin and therefore to store more fat. It causes free radical damage of cells, to the inner walls of arteries and veins leading to lethargy, wrinkles (yes, age is simply the accumulation of toxins), fatigue, obesity and more. To help alkalinise, put lemon in your water. Use it with a tiny bit of better quality salt like Himalayan and good oil for salad dressing. Try sprouted wheat breads and wheatgrass juices. Keep salad handy at all times.

The following are all acid addictions: caffeine, alcohol, drugs, and whites. Avoid wheat products, bread, rice, sugar and potatoes because they spike your blood sugar; also nicotine and vinegar. Reduce animal flesh and dairy products.

Get your enzymes from raw foods: eat green veg or salad every day.

Combining foods in certain ways, for example not having carbs with protein, aids digestion. Green salad ought to be eaten with carbs, protein or fat (fats inhibit the digestion of protein; salad will offset this). Fruits are best eaten alone on an empty stomach. Don't drink with or immediately following a meal; finish drinking water thirty minutes before meals and wait thirty minutes after before drinking again. Drinking before helps fill you up, and not drinking during aids digestion.

When I help clients with weight issues, I ask if they want a quick fix or an ongoing lifestyle change that will be more effective long-term. As a hypnotherapist, I can motivate clients in any way they choose, but my ethos and holistic background influence me to guide them towards the deeper changes that they can live with permanently. Although it's not always easy to gather feedback, I have noticed that the clients, who do take that advice, even if they are only able to make small changes at a time, are the ones who enjoy the longer-term results.

Eating consciously also helps, and it is a great opportunity to practice mindfulness. Eliminate all distractions, make a ritual of both cooking and eating. Preparing food you love is just another way of giving to yourself and thus boosting your self-esteem.

My porridge became famous during my yoga-teacher training at my very favourite retreat here in Scotland, Anam Cara. During a five-day juicing detox I attended there, Margaret, our facilitator, explained about putting love into the juice we were preparing, and sipping in silence with great appreciation. Believe me, after a day or two of no other food, that wasn't hard to do! I later adapted that idea to the porridge. Our guru, Daizan began with meditation at 5 a.m. each day, and by breakfast time, we were ravenous. So I'd prepare the night before, singing my little song into the pot as I stirred: "This is the porridge of love, baby, this is the porridge of joy, this is the porridge of peace." The desired state is added as an ingredient, just like infusing your drinking water with love – you will taste the difference!

Eat consciously and prepare with love!

Eating consciously means preparing with love, sitting comfortably; taking small bites, chewing thoroughly, savouring the flavour, respecting the effort, the ingredients and the company.

I am not a nutritionist; I am just sharing ideas that have helped me and I encourage you to:

Learn about nutrition: about what kind of fuel your body needs for optimum energy and vitality.

Movement

It may be true that we are exercising more than we did in the 80s; there certainly seem to be more gyms and personal trainers than twenty years ago, but are we moving more? How many of us are desk-bound and working horrendous hours? Even young kids are suffering bad posture through overuse of computers, and few of us actually use the full range of movement the human body was designed for. When the body gets out of alignment like that and we fail to exercise and build the muscles that support its structure, it paves the way for challenges with balance, metabolism, sight, even fertility and many other fundamental biological processes.

Exercise is just learning to love moving ourselves.

So what to do? Whether you are already exercising or not, you need to move yourself more. Get up frequently and shake your booty, put on your favourite music and dance, go up and down the stairs, do some housework every night. Walk the dog more. Play with the kids, the cat, the mother-in-law or somebody a whole lot more exciting in the evenings. Anything rather than sedentary activities like watching television. I strongly recommend yoga:

"Yoga is first and foremost a science of self-realisation. Its concern is spiritual practice and serving the person's spiritual evolution mainly through meditation. Yoga provides the key to all spiritual development that comprises gaining knowledge of our true nature beyond time, space, death and suffering." Seda Shambhavi Kervanogiu

Not too fussed about your spiritual evolution? I hear you. Then try this on: compare the physiques of most yoga practitioners to those of the general population. Got it? So whether you look at it from a shallow or a deep perspective, yoga is good for you, even home practice. Indeed, most forms of fitness are entirely doable at home these days. How far you take things is up to you. This isn't an exercise book, but if you are uncomfortable in your own skin, doing something about the physical side of things is often the easiest place to start.

This is what happened with Eileen, a client of mine, way back in my fitness trainer days. Eileen had two lovely dogs and lived out of the city. When we first met I visited her at home and wasn't even allowed to say the word "gym." Eileen wanted to shed a little weight and tone up, so it was time for her and the dogs to get fit. The four of us went power walking for just over a year and progressed to using basic equipment and body weight. That year set her up. Looking positively statuesque, toned, with a beautifully cut bicep, Eileen had lost fat and gained muscle. During that time her self-confidence rose, and she thrilled in shopping for clothes, as everything looked so good on her. She was so proud when she went on a girly holiday: 'I didn't cover myself up – I have a bikini body!'

We lost touch, and when we re-connected some years later she was a six-day-a-week gym bunny training for the New York marathon. I couldn't believe I was talking to the same woman. We re-connected for a third time on a return flight from Turkey where I had just completed the first draft of this book and she was returning from a yoga retreat. Our relationship had spanned nearly twenty years by then. We met up for coffee so I could ask permission to share her story.

The keenest question on my lips was what had been the turning point for her. I knew meeting me had been pivotal, but I wanted to know about the inner experience. Initially, she said, it was the realisation that: "Wow, this is cool, I like feeling like this" Secondly, after believing as a child that she would not amount to much, it was discovering that she could train and achieve something to feel proud of. Her self-esteem grew and grew. She accepted a job as editor of a golf magazine, despite, as she told me, "Never having swung a golf bat," something she would never have considered before mastering her body.

The story has a lovely ending in that Eileen is not only about to marry the man of her dreams, but runs a successful home boarding business for very happy and very fit dogs. When I asked her the question "Would you say you are being the 'me you want to be'?" she answered with an emphatic YES!

Begin with the kind of exercise that will work in your life, but know that you can easily make time to move more.

How are you treating your Temple?

If you are physically fit, you can react better to stress, depression and indeed any of the curve balls life tends to throw.

Regular exercise will reduce the risk of premature death by 40 percent – that means more fun, more joy, more whatever it is you want more of before you die. It activates the parasympathetic nervous system and lowers the blood pressure, so it is relaxing. It will improve cardiovascular functioning and muscle tone, thus preventing wear and tear of joints, leaving you buff and flexible! It increases the intake of oxygen, and since oxygen is the fuel of metabolism, you'll burn more calories, and each breath you take will be more efficient.

The main thing to target is aerobic exercise, as improved stamina will serve you well when it comes to facing any kind of pressure. Stamina is improved by swimming, cycling, running, jogging, and brisk walking. Strength is improved by lifting weights, especially your body weight. Flexibility is key: stretch regularly or practice yoga. Stretching reduces tension in muscles, can be done in a few minutes and will have an immediate effect on your sense of wellbeing.

I read a great book called Younger by Next Year: Live Strong, Fit, and Sexy – Until You're 80 and Beyond by Chris Crowley and Henry S. Lodge. The authors challenge the widely held belief that you hit a certain age, go over the hill, and face the slow downhill trundle through degenerating health, to disease and death. They argue, backed by solid research, that, to the contrary, you can retain the fitness and health achieved in your later years and stay fit and healthy until you die. In other words, stay on a plateau until game over.

So it doesn't matter what age you are; you can improve things now and retain the benefits of those changes through to a robust old age. Personally, I can't count the number of times I've thought, "Oh well, that's it, I've done it now," or "Oh, that will be the end of that," then made some changes and become amazed at the sheer healing ability of my own body and mind. For me, the two go hand in hand: if I eat and exercise properly, my mind will be my friend. So, find the time to exercise!

"They" say to try a minimum of two 20-minute exercise sessions per week, but three 30-minute workouts are better, and five better still. Personally, I exercise most days. Crowley and Lodge say the one thing that can trick your body into believing it is younger is to make it produce human growth hormone, which you can achieve by exercising really hard. Whatever age or level you are at:

Choose an aerobic exercise that you enjoy.

Pick the same time every day / week.

Gradually increase exercise intensity and duration.

Something is better than nothing – up to you how far you go.

Finding an exercise partner or trainer can help get you started.

Learn to move yourself and keep moving: what kind of exercise could you really enjoy?

You need to master your body on several levels, how you move it, how you water and fuel it, and also through the chemicals you encourage it to produce.

Physiological State

Think of it like this: your brain is just a computer, albeit the most highly efficient one on the planet. It keeps the organic superstructure that is your body ticking over in good health.

Your body is a chemical factory, one that can produce highs and lows according to the messages it receives from the brain.

Your mind is a thought-producing machine. The mind produces thoughts, and will do so till the day you die; it's an eternal cycle. That's its job. You may not be entirely in charge of which thoughts come up, and for sure some are just debris from the information highway, but you certainly are in charge of which thoughts you stay with and subsequently of the chemicals your brain tells your body to produce.

Your bodily needs affect your physiological state. If you are tired, hungry, thirsty, or ill, you simply will not feel good; you will not be in a good state. At the same time, your physiological state affects your physical body. Remain in a less-than-ideal state for too long and the effects will be detrimental.

Being in a detrimental state, of course, affects your thinking and your feelings. It can cause you to say nasty things to yourself, so that you end up negatively hypnotising yourself and thus sabotaging your good efforts. Then your amazing chemical factory will not be instructed to produce the right cocktail for optimum performance and wellbeing.

Conversely the right mind-set can change your physiology in a positive way. The placebo, which, by the way, is the most successful drug on the planet, proves this.

So certainly your physiological state includes your mental and emotional bodies, but there is plenty you can do about your state from the purely physical. For instance, what state are you in right now? Are you in the best state for this reading, for learning, for relaxing? It's actually your choice. What do you need to get there? Better light, another chair, better posture? Do you need to clean your specs, to drink, eat, or move? If you want to feel calm, simply take a few breaths, and practice one of the exercises included in the Resources and Recordings. Want to let go of frustration, anger or fear? Walk up a hill; run with the dog; move around; visit the nearest swimming pool, sauna or steam room. Want to feel excited? Stand up, play music, dance, sing.

A client of mine, Dereck, had been depressed for years – I mean well over a decade, if not two. During one of our Skype sessions, he reluctantly agreed that whatever he had been practicing that week had left him feeling good. Well, of course, who jumped into my head but James Brown:

I feel good!

Music is a great state-changer; so is dancing around to your favourite track or singing silly songs that you make up yourself, especially about your own situation.

Remember Muhammad Ali: *"Float like a butterfly, sting like a bee."*

Lots of athletes do that. Ever watched the pre-race theatre during the Olympics? Did you see Usain Bolt's salute? Some of you may even remember Churchill's V for victory. What about a simple thumbs-up, or punching the air? Just giving yourself a shake can help change your state. Make up your own move or dance! Why not do it right now?

Whatever you do, let's not pretend you are not in control. Have you ever been ill, moping around not able to get out of bed, when suddenly an unexpected visitor shows up whom under no circumstances you'll allow to see you like that? Your brain, the computer, tells your body, the chemical factory: "Oh, shit, need to step into action here – hit me with the adrenalin, please."

And while you get your sorry ass into the shower and start shaking it around a little, your body responds: "At last, movement – let's give her a little feel-good shot of endorphins."

So you put on a little slap, put on your best 'phoney' smile and before you know it, you are engaged! In the moment! The unwelcome visitor leaves, and guess what? You got it: you miraculously feel better...

Ever seen a slovenly teen perk up at the sight, thought, never mind the appearance, of a peer of the opposite sex? Mmmmm, yes - so DON'T TELL ME you're not in charge of your state!

Why, I've helped some clients move on from what were deep-seated habitual behaviours like nail-biting, hair pulling and twitching – in some cases habits that had lasted over fifty years. First I'd tell them they were lying when they said they couldn't help it. Then, when they looked at me incredulously, I would fish around for times when they didn't do it, for example while having hot, passionate sex! Well, if you can desist then, you really can't say you can't help it, can you? You know what I'm talking about...you choose!

Change your state again, again and again!

Every day, wake up and decide what state you choose to be in for the day. You're in charge. Then simply remember how it is to feel that way. If you don't know, pretend, imagine, or fake it till you make it! You will soon start to believe it at a cellular level and therefore become it.

Physiology is key!

Let me put it another way. You don't get to feel like a world-class boxing champ by sitting with your shoulders slumped, head drooped, telling yourself it's a waste of time anyway. You get up, move around, breathe deep, shake your ass and either remember or imagine good stuff like first kisses, knowing glances, great sex, wetting yourself laughing, fun times in the sun and beautiful rainbows – do it and get into the state you choose to be in! The reason thinking about good times we've had makes us feel so good is that the subconscious mind doesn't know the difference between imagination and reality. That's why this stuff really works. If you can imagine it, you can be it – simple as that!

The imagination is where you create your reality.

Try this: close your eyes and remember your first romantic kiss... nice? Perhaps not, but sure you remembered it, including the accompanying feelings. Now...

Imagine you are on a long, carefree Mediterranean holiday, living in an old rustic farmhouse situated in its own orchard.

Late one afternoon, you wander into the cool kitchen to prepare the evening drinks.

On the big wooden table there's a huge bowl of lemons you'd taken from the tree earlier in the day. Ripe and ready, all shades of yellow and green.

Reach over and pick the juiciest lemon, feeling the dimpled peel as you bring it to the chopping board. Already you can smell the lemony smell.

With a sharp knife, you slice it open, and as the juice sprays your face, you really smell the tangy lemony smell and your mouth begins to water in anticipation of the taste...

You bring it to your mouth unable to resist tasting that lovely juicy lemon.

Are you salivating? See where I am going with this? The unconscious reacts to imagination and memory in the same ways it reacts to reality. What about playing the music that reminds you of the time that...the friend that...the holiday that...yes, it takes you right back there, it changes your state, so take charge!

Begin NOW: be with what is. Maybe you cannot control other people or certain circumstances, but you can choose your state day-by-day, minute-by-minute!

Breathing, drinking, eating and moving with consciousness is the base line of everything that follows and will absolutely affect your physiological state. To keep yourself in peak physiological state, go into the realm of imagination and keep going there until it becomes your reality. Set up lots of reminders, many times every single day, to take the small steps suggested in the follow up emails that will give you results in less than a month.

The next thing we'll look at is the mind. Your mind. After all, that is what this is all about: your mind, your body, your thoughts, your feelings, and your initiation to the self.

You're doing great!

Chapter 3

MASTERING THE MIND

Ancient Egyptian would-be initiates attained mastery of the mind and body before entering the King's Chamber for three days without food and water, since failure meant certain death.

You too can learn to detach from and master your thoughts.

You are not your thoughts...

Learn Meditation and Mindfulness

You are not your thoughts, although it can sometimes seem that way when they apparently take over and control you. The antidote is meditation. Without a shadow of a doubt, meditation is the best way to still the mind.

The benefits of meditation have been known to man for thousands of years. Initiates to the priesthood in ancient Egypt and yogis in India could survive being shut in initiation chambers for long periods due to the strength of their practice. That very same practice can equip you for the stresses and strains of modern living.

Meditation not only leads to mastery of the mind, but also to mastery of the chemical factory that is your body. This can be seen in all the physiological measurements of stress, measurements, which indicate strongly that meditation reduces stress, strengthens the immune system and helps the body's natural healing process. By mastering these things, you become better able to control your emotions and inner nature. This is true for all of us, not just the gurus amongst us. Although 'guru got it all together' can seem at the opposite end of the spectrum from where you currently are.

When you are in pain, are feeling ashamed, unworthy or pulling your hair out by the roots, unable to quell the ranting rage in your head or the dull ache in your heart, the suggestion to meditate may seem trite or even patronising. Meditation can seem like a pastime for those with nothing better to do, or perhaps an invitation to sandal-wearing escapism.

However, when I say meditation, I'm talking in the very simplest sense; all I mean is taking time to stop, find a quiet place within, and staying there in silence, allowing the chatter of the mind to subside. Try it: thirty seconds is enough to begin! The step-by-step instructions are coming up. So many of my clients and students say they have not meditated before, not even had the desire to be alone, and really don't know where to start. Others are already virtuosos, much more disciplined in their practice than I'll ever be. Wherever you are, take this opportunity to establish or re-establish a practice.

Over the years, the feedback I have received from those who have embraced meditation in their lives, including myself, is that one day you just notice the mental torture has stopped. Shit still happens of course, but now you know how to get off of the merry go round. You have a tool, which produces a greater level of stillness on a daily basis.

So if you'd like to permanently see the end of fretting, iffing, butting and shoulding all over yourself, lock the door and switch the phone off right now. Take note of how you feel before so you can compare it to how you feel after. I'll guide you through the rest – just go to the link in the Resources and Recordings. Then make a resolution to build up to between ten to thirty minutes' practice over the next month. I've provided the tools, you've nothing else to do, so treat it as an experiment. After twenty-one days, the habit will become unconscious and I'll bet my shirt you notice the benefits!

Whatever happens during practice is good. You did it, and that's enough for now; relaxation will come eventually. Sometimes it takes several practice sessions to even become aware of the effects; at first you may not be sure what to look for. Keep going; practice is the key. The practice in itself may not be relaxing or restful, however, it will bring improvements that paradoxically allow you to be more relaxed in your life. Meditation is a skill, and like any skill, the more you practice, the better you will become. Without practice, you will not improve. To benefit, you must actually do it. An athlete doesn't become a champion without training, and you won't master anything without practice. It takes both action and effort to evolve the discipline of practice. By practicing you will change, you will reset your computer to reduce anxiety about, and increase quality of performance in, everything in life. Focus, sustained attention and cognitive ability, will improve – which simply means you will be here, be present. How many times have you missed a really great moment because your head was in the clouds – this is the antidote!

I was introduced to meditation in 1987 when my mother dragged me along to a transcendental meditation class. It was during the early days of my recovery from heroin addiction when I didn't even want to leave my room. I remember steeling myself to walk the fifty yards to the paper shop. I counted the sapling larch on the way, wondering at the ugliness of their grey supports with the dull metal straps, yet the truth is I needed something like that myself. It was terrifying just walking down the street. I wasn't even aware that I had become numb to life, never mind having a clue what to do about it. I managed to occupy the galloping rant in my brain with studying. I pacified the cravings with the fat and sugar in the "Aberdeen roll" I set out every day to buy. Meditation, well, I'm not even certain I can remember doing it that first three years. I did though, and once my body found its fitness again and the chemical rampage began to settle down I did notice a growing calm. Then one day I noticed the buds on one of those larch and realised life could renew itself and so could I. Awareness kind of crept up on me after that, although believe me there have been many times when I wished I could put it back!

So meditation wakes you up – takes you out of whatever illusion you pretend is reality, but there's more, much, much more.

Other Benefits of Meditation

Meditating makes you younger. Short term meditators test physiologically five years younger than their non-meditating counterparts. Those practicing for five years test twelve years younger and some subjects tested, had a biological age twenty-seven years younger than their chronological age. When meditation is introduced to elderly people, they show numerous beneficial changes, including ultimately living longer and those benefits endure when tested more than ten years later!

Dan Buettner, author of The Blue Zones and researcher into longevity hotspots around the world, suggests small lifestyle changes can add up to ten years to most people's lives. He says ageing is ten percent genetic and ninety percent lifestyle and that having mechanisms to shed stress, like prayer and meditation, is of high importance in the longevity hotspots he studied, and a major factor in long-term health and ageing.

Meditation is fast becoming the treatment of choice for chronic pain, which has fantastic implications for medication use. Up to fifty percent of people with chronic pain have depression, and meditation trains the brain to be more focused on the present and therefore spend less time anticipating future negative events, which is one of the hallmarks of depression. This focus on the present may be why meditation is effective at reducing the recurrence of depression, which makes chronic pain considerably worse. In fact, studies have shown that mindfulness and meditation have proved as effective as maintenance anti-depressants in preventing a relapse, and were even more effective in enhancing people's quality of life. Even weekly meditation lessons, backed by short daily practice improves quality of sleep and lowers feelings of stress. Having facilitated meditation and relaxation classes since 2001, I have seen this for myself. If there is one universal piece of feedback from my classes and recordings it is: "What a great night's sleep I had," and that's after just one time! Yes, improvements are shown in just one day, and the longer you practice, the better you become. Research shows that positive personality growth and psychological benefits increase with experience, improving overall self-esteem, feelings of worthiness, benevolence, and self-acceptance. It is really good for you – so get going!

Practicing meditation and mindfulness in your daily life raises your self-awareness to the level where you can truly master yourself. It can help you choose how you spend your moments and your days. Help you wake up with more energy, a more positive attitude and provide you with an openness that allows you to observe yourself, everything around you and the flow of life. The more you connect with that energy, the better able you are to make the right decision in the right timing.

Am I saying you have to meditate? No, I am saying that you have to sit still long enough to hear the answers. Meditation is just a way of making yourself do so.

You also need to be aware of what you say to yourself outside of practice. Consider this:

"The mind and body are the same system. Every cell is eavesdropping on your internal dialogue." Deepak Chopra

The Power of Thought and the Truth about the Subconscious Mind

What you say to yourself is crucial. If you have a negative voice inside your head which likes to nag and scold, there is absolutely no point in doing any of this, as self-sabotage by negative hypnosis will make your inner scolding become a self-fulfilling prophecy. If, for instance, you eat chocolate while telling yourself it will go "straight to the hips," that is surely where it will go.

Thinking is just a subtle form of hearing.

Let's look at the scientific backup we have for claiming that what we say to ourselves is crucial.

Thirty years ago someone produced a survey claiming stress had no role in cancer. The fantastic thing about this survey was that it produced such a tremendous backlash that we now have hundreds of studies showing us how the mind affects our physiology. Research that proves your immune cells are constantly eavesdropping on your inner dialogue, so that when they hear "I'm fed up," "I don't like my job," or "I can't bear another day like this," they soon start to feel the same. Let's face it: wouldn't you, when exposed to negativity all day? The next thing you know, your immune cells start to communicate in the same way:

"Can't be bothered fighting that invader cell." "Not interested in trying anymore." And so on...

By contrast, words (therefore thoughts, chemicals and feelings) like: "Life's great," "I'm so excited about the future," and "I'm totally awesome" attract a similar response from your cells:

"Oh, it looks as if that cell over there is about to alter its genetic code. I'll just pop over and give it a gentle reminder..." NUDGE!

In the same way, your T-cells can tell your B-cells to rev up and go into battle. So what you say to yourself is VITAL. Your inner dialogue is absolutely crucial to your wellbeing and I cannot stress that enough. Hence, from the mistress of the affirmation:

"Every thought we think is creating our future." Louise Hay

Affirmations

So, how do YOU speak to yourself: body, mind, soul, energetic being, and portion of the cosmos?

Are you repeating words of the past, echoes from childhood? Do you scold yourself, or are you kind and gentle with yourself as you would be with a dear friend? Think about it, and think about how you could be encouraging yourself. One way of encouraging yourself is by using affirmations. Most of us have probably spent a large part of our lives doing negative hypnosis or affirmations, so why not go the other way for a while?

I love the way Louise Hay in You Can Heal Your Life offers: "I love myself." OK, if it feels all wrong or just a bit phony, change it to: "I'm willing to learn to love myself." Feel easier? In other words, be gentle with yourself as you learn these new skills.

If this is more your style, though, try: "Even though I am totally crap in social situations, I totally love and accept myself." Go for that and see how it affects your daily life.

Or courtesy of the barefoot doctor: "It's OK to mentally beat myself up so long as I am enjoying it, and either way I am still not a bad chappy. In fact, I scrub up pretty well and can even be delectably dapper and lots of fun on a good day." In other words, make it real for you!

Another method is to insert your name and use three different pronouns: "I, Vicki, am financially secure, fantastically fit, and living life to the full."

"She, Vicki, is financially secure, fantastically fit and living life to the full."

"You, Vicki, are financially secure, fantastically fit, and living life to the full."

This would have been how you were originally programmed, by telling yourself limiting or negative ideas, being told them by others and overhearing them discussed by others, so challenge them on those three levels.

Get Excited!

Affirmations can be lots of fun, yet they always fell a bit flat for me when served up cold like that. Then I heard Tony Robbins talk about getting excited – his talks are all about getting excited, and I'm all for that!

Think about it: someone suffering post-traumatic stress disorder has an imprint on their mind because they've witnessed a horrible event while in fight-or-flight mode – in other words, while excited. This is why the image sticks. So reverse it and realise how powerful your affirmations and amazing visuals can become if you are physically excited as you play them, i.e. meticulously choose your best state before putting your order in with the cosmos.

I had great fun after someone told me about a lady they knew who had been singing in the shower to lose weight. It was all about self-acceptance: "I love my curvy ass" and "my glorious abundant boobs." A few of my weight-loss clients experimented and, yes, it worked. One client, who was thinking her other half must be fancying a gorgeous celeb instead of her, tried it too. I won't say what she was singing, but suffice to say they ended up in the Caribbean on a romantic holiday for two!

Remember Dereck in the last chapter:

I feel good!

So sing, dance, jog, jump up and down and chant your lungs out, let yourself feel those good feelings. In other words, get excited about this new life you're creating!

If you were your own best friend and had to find something complimentary to say about yourself, you would find something: eyes; turn of the ankle; hair; skin; smile. Start with that. I'm sure there are lots of lovable things about you, but the trick is for YOU to find some. If not, ask your best friend and begin from there.

Find words that will really work for you. State in positive terms, in **your** language, what you would **really** say in the privacy of your own home, in the way that you would **actually** say it. Then shout it, sing it, or dance it! Find occasions during the day when you can repeat those words ritualistically, maybe during or after the relaxation techniques you are practicing. The point is to change your physiology while repeating your affirmations. It is not the same as recounting the shopping list for Tesco. This is your shopping list to the cosmos – so get passionate!

Pattern Interrupt

Adding new and exciting material is also a great way of moving beyond the voices of the past. In fact, putting a different spin on things can help you get rid of stubborn negative thoughts from the present too.

You can change the character of the voice inside your head. "That was stupid" doesn't sound quite so harsh murmured in the sexy tones of Marilyn Monroe; nor, "You'll never amount to anything" a la Mickey Mouse. How about Arnold Schwarzenegger doing, "Do you really need that cheesecake?" It can be any character you like, because guess what – you're the director! You can tell yourself anything, spin your internal dialogue any way you choose. No one else knows what's going on in your head. No one knows whether you're telling yourself you are an amazing, gorgeous love god or goddess, or giving yourself a mental spanking the Marquis de Sade would be proud of, only you (and that includes the universe) will hear it, and if you don't act on it, the universe will. In the end, your beliefs are yours. I realised early on I could believe whatever I liked, so I chose those beliefs that served me best.

You can use exactly the same technique to cope with the type of people, who bleat on in a predictable fashion. See them as acting a role you have created for them – 'grumpy git,' 'negative Ned,' 'winging Wilma,' and 'projecting Paula,' cast them in full caricature, and soon you will see the funny side. Once they have delivered their oh-so-predictable lines just say: "Cut, in the can," laugh, and let it go.

Keeping an eye on your negative inner dialogue and creating new, helpful, words will set you in the direction you intend to travel. Again, this is not about endlessly reciting affirmations in a drone-like fashion. We don't need to work that hard to try to 'fix' or 'heal' things. Don't get stuck in your own words or trance. Morph into the right state, be fabulously grateful for what you have right now and ask if there are any shifts you need to make. In fact continually ask questions and through the practice of meditation and mindfulness you will have the calm and the awareness to hear the answers. You will have made the connection with the still voice within that leads you to the wisdom of your heart and soul. Away from the past and into the now.

If that hasn't convinced you, nothing ever will. Just try it. Give me those twenty-one days!

Rome wasn't built in one day, begin now – do the best you can!

Before we leave the subject of mind, I'd like to talk a little about the hypnotherapist's favourite tool – the subconscious mind.

Subconscious v Unconscious

The mind stores all memories from past, present and perhaps even the future. It works in mysterious ways, is connected deeply to the collective unconsciousness as described by Carl Jung, and links each and every one of us to the creative source of power, to the cosmos itself. In psychotherapy, we use the word unconscious to describe that part of our consciousness that can 'never' be reached, and the subconscious as that part that we can become aware of and work with.

The subconscious mind reacts to imagination and memory in the same ways it reacts to reality; it simply cannot tell the difference – remember the first kiss, slicing the lemon, the nostalgic music from Chapter Two? You experienced all the feelings (chemicals) as if you were actually there.

The subconscious mind is hugely obedient; in fact, it is your loyal servant and will most definitely create upon the stage of your life the movie you play in your mind. This happens whether you fuel it with negative hypnosis and devices of self-sabotage or beautiful images and incantations. So whether you frolic in fantasy or delve in despair, your dreams will come true, so choose them well. YOU are most definitely the one in control, and as master chef, YOU decide what ingredients to put in the cauldron, or, since the physicists came on board, the quantum soup!

So tell yourself you are a god or goddess walking the earth attracting love, abundance, incredible beings and amazing experiences into your reality. And tell yourself how well you are doing with every little thing. Do it for twenty-one days and let me know whether I am right or not. You decide which method works best.

Here's something else to take note of – what happens if I ask you not to think of a pink elephant? A pink elephant wearing a blue tutu and orange wig, tap-dancing on the table – exactly. Let me explain:

The subconscious mind doesn't hear the word "NO." It will not recognise negatives. That is simply the way it operates; it's a fact. So when I say: Do not think of a pink elephant, you have no choice but to think of one. So there's no point in nutting yourself (I will not stress, I will not smoke, I will not eat sweeties). You need to tell the subconscious mind, your loyal servant, the cosmic dinner lady or the genie in the magic lamp, what you do want. What you want instead, your desired outcome, your goal. You need to picture it.

The subconscious mind is hugely visual – remember the wig wearing, tap dancing pink elephant. The subconscious loves symbols and metaphors, far prefers them to words, in fact, it needs symbolic communication to understand what you want to achieve so you'll feel more compelled and motivated if you create an even bigger, brighter and more exciting picture, a more powerful vision. Try it and see.

This works in reverse too. It is how my clients terrorise themselves into a quivering wreck at the mere thought of public speaking, a trip to the supermarket or catching sight of a ginormous being dressed in a yellow and black suit with a pointy weapon in its tail. Yes they make huge terrifying pictures of it. In NLP we use this info to help as it always works like this: create the picture, tell yourself something about the picture (negative hypnosis) and experience all the exciting chemicals associated with the sheer panic you have just created, which in the case of wasp phobia, you can use to power yourself around the lawn at the garden party screaming at the top of your lungs. Great fun!

If you add to the above, the fact that the subconscious mind operates much better when plied with great cocktails of chemicals and hormones (preferably produced by the chemical factory that is your body, managed by the computer that is your brain and directed by the amazing being that is YOU!), you can see why the above scenario can become a raging phobia. Equally, you can use these facts to get into and stay in that ZONE where life is flowing and synchronicities are abounding. Get and stay in peak state.

So your subconscious mind works in pictures, deletes all negatives yet hears and obeys everything you say, if that is not enough for you, and just to add a little icing on the cake – it also has a great sense of humour! I'll let you discover that one for yourself.

The subconscious mind also provides an early warning system, both clues to what is next and what needs looked at. It sends you really cool messages called dreams and in fact will happily entertain you nightly with person-alised movies. It also sends you 'symptoms' and messages via your body to let you know that something needs attention. This marvellous 'entity' is in communication with you all the time – so watch what you are saying back!

Now that you have mastered your mind, you can master your emotions in a similar way: 'Mastering the Emotions' is the next chapter.

Chapter 4

MASTERING THE EMOTIONS

The ancient Egyptians used the power of their emotions to take them to a higher level of being.

You too can learn to master your emotions and use the energy thus released to jump out of fear and into alignment with the synchronous flow of the cosmos.

You are not your emotions…

Sitting with the Emotions

You too can learn to be at one with your emotions.

In the temple schools, neophytes would experience each emotion as it naturally arose. Once comfortable with that, they'd practice summoning each emotion at will, then they would move from one emotion to the next, finally learning to use the emotions as a platform to the spiritual realms. In this learning they realised that they could master their emotions, and therefore their state.

When you think about it, it makes perfect sense. Everything is energy: hurt, jealousy, anger – all just energy. They are e-motions, that same energy in motion that the ancients used to connect with spirit. When you try to dam up or deny emotion, there is no motion and therefore no growth. On the other hand, when you allow and encourage the e-motion, you release stuck energy, you create a space, a vacuum, an opportunity to grow. Nature abhors a vacuum and sucks in new energy. Accompany that natural flow with intent to use that energy, to e-mote all that you desire, all that you dream and all that you truly deserve. All that is available and waiting for you on this beautiful planet.

"Everything is energy and that's all there is to it. Match the frequency of the reality you want and you cannot help but get that reality. It can be no other way. This is not philosophy. This is physics." Albert Einstein

Perhaps it sounds like a tall order, but I'll show you exactly how to master your emotions with great simplicity. Being a therapist, helping others doing exactly that, albeit couched in different terms, has given me great satisfaction over the years, so it is a joy to share it with you now.

Typically a client arrives, controlled by how they are feeling, believing that is how they ARE. In fact, they've been feeling that way for so long, they believe it is WHO they are, and that they have no power to change it. They'll have their own particular theory, perhaps one of their parents was that way, so they think it's genetic, or they feel it was caused by a series of events or unfortunate circumstances out of their control. It is an honour and a joy to watch them go through the process that turns their pain around, sometimes instant and magical, and at other times beginning with doubts:

"I've tried everything else, so I thought I would give hypnosis a go."

"Do you have to believe in it?"

Clients can resist the work, resist the change at first, but eventually we find an area where they become willing to at least experiment. They experience one or two instances where it does work, then, eureka! The blossoming when they realise things can change, they can let go, things can be different, is wonderful. A whole new world opens up for them, and they feel like new person, free to live and love and enjoy a great quality of life.

I'd like to offer you that same freedom through a meditation that was given to me by Willaru, a Master from the Andean Mystery School.

Present Moment Emotions

I went to Peru after discovering my husband had fallen in love with a young Russian woman while working in Kazakhstan. I felt like my world had ended. After things erupted and he went back there, I was concerned regarding what I would do when he came home again. The fighting had been bitter and I knew we couldn't stand another four weeks like that. Then out of the blue, in popped an invitation for a spiritual journey to Peru from a beautiful sister and fellow seeker, a woman who has influenced my life in many ways, Maggie Erotokritou. There were two places left, and we grabbed them. One of many synchronicities that have blessed my life.

Two days after my then-husband returned home, I walked out the door leaving everything I knew and loved. Twelve years of being a family, just the three of us, the animals, baking bread, weekend-long stay-overs, outdoor pursuits and cosy fires. I was broken. I stopped by the home of a very dear friend on the way to the airport: "How can I do it, how can I leave?" She put her arm around me and asked me to look at my feet. I did. Now, she said, put one foot in front of the other. I did. I walked with tears in every part of my being. For many of the days that followed, that was all I could do, put one foot in front of the other. I'll never forget her words nor the love she showed me that day.

Next thing I knew, I was in Cuzco chewing on coca leaves, my soul now crying to the tune of the panpipes. Peru was an amazing experience in every way. How odd it was to be, for the first time in my life, the 'woman who cried.' I'd facilitated many groups by then and helped people through their pain, but this was the first time I'd stood in their shoes. In front of a group of twenty-seven spiritual seekers, I cried and cried and cried. I was so used to being the strongest, bravest, most together person in groups, the oldest and toughest in my family, yet now the tears would only switch off long enough for me to eat my evening meal. I was so hungry by then, but by the last mouthful, I'd be off again.

Eventually I asked for help. Willaru's Golden Flame in the Temple of the

Heart, which you can find in the Resources and Recordings, has not only saved me from myself and what seemed like overwhelming and uncontrollable emotions, but has given me a connection to myself that provides me with all the answers I'll ever need. I thank you, Willaru, from the bottom of my heart.

Learning to Let Go

What Willaru taught was acknowledging, accepting and being with what is. You need to also let go of what isn't, that is, your dramas and the stories you tell yourself which perpetuate the unhealthy feelings. Golden Flame is the best tool that I have ever found for letting go and creating new energy to move forward in life.

There are other ways, of course. You can pummel a cushion or writhe on the floor, but that's a bit California for a proper Scottish lass like me. Perhaps if you pay enough, you can scream at your therapist. I felt like doing that once: she told me I had to let go and when I asked her how, she said, "Whatever feels right for you," or some other person-centred junket meaning she couldn't tell me. I asked a teacher, and she couldn't tell me either. She gave me a metaphor about a man who was holding onto a rope for dear life. His guardian angel eventually persuaded him to let go and he found that his feet had been on the ground the whole time. I got it, but I still had no clue where the rope was or what to do with huge waves of emotions washing over me. So Willaru had given me the practical key. I practiced the Golden Flame in the Temple of the Heart and kept on practicing – it works! Several years later when I attended a seminar – 'Helping clients tolerate difficult emotions' I received the theory.

It goes like this: when an escalating emotion begins to feel so uncomfortable that you can't bear the thought of the suffering any longer, you jump off the mountain into self-defeating behaviours like eating, drinking, and preoccupying yourself with work, sex or rock and roll. Thus you never get to the peak of the emotion so it cannot find its natural resolution. Such a pity when you were so near the top anyway.

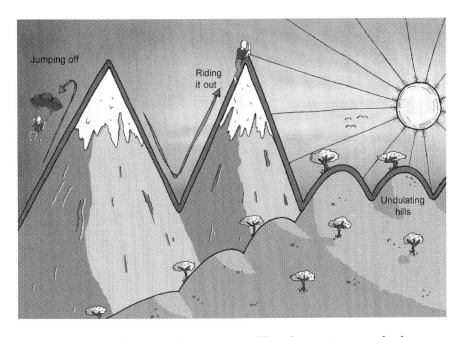

If you were to ride it out, first you would realise it is not as bad as you anticipated. Sitting in your power with an emotion is a whole different ballgame from being overpowered by it. You find it will arise and pass, just as your thoughts do in meditation. Sometimes another emotion does appear in its place, but just repeat the process and keep going until you are left with that feeling of calm when the roller coaster dies down. You will always feel emotions; it is part of being human, but instead of having mad peaks and troughs, you can have gentle undulating hills and dales.

At the time I received the Golden Flame in the Temple of the Heart from Willaru, I thought the tears would never end. Eventually they did, but I wish I'd known this then – an emotion only lasts sixteen to twenty seconds: yes, that's all!

I've asked clients many times how long they thought an emotion lasted, and their answers vary from a minute to years. It seems longer because we try to avoid feeling the feelings. In fact, we usually do the opposite to what would actually help us! The truth is, the more you resist anything, the more it will persist. It doesn't matter how many times you jump off of the mountain or bury your head in the sand: the same emotion will keep recurring until you face it, until you use the energy in motion to propel you through the changes needed in your life. This is because whatever you resist or push against simply persists and pushes back in equal measure. So instead, transform resistance into acceptance and remind yourself:

Que sera, sera. Whatever will be, will be.

So accept where you are right now, do the work of the Temple of the Heart: Golden Flame to let go and Looking Within to observe and find your true needs moment to moment. If you don't let go you will stay stuck, and if you don't make it your business to get what you need, it will be impossible to attract what you want, and that's where you're going, moving towards living the life of your dreams, so...

Let go, take action on your needs and give yourself your heart's desire.

Meeting Your Own Needs

In the end there is no option but to take responsibility for your own needs. That doesn't mean being totally self-centred and irresponsible, although prioritising yourself may make you feel like that at first since many of us were taught that it was selfish to do so. However, the truth is, we all have needs, ALL of the time; it is part of being human.

You have needs all the way up from your requirement for fresh air, water and food – the first three things the body dies without. You also need shelter, warmth, rest, physical safety and human contact. You need good relationships with others and with yourself. A sense of purpose and a sense of belonging. You need predictability and stability as well as stimulation, excitement and adventure. You need to be appreciated and to have a sense that in some way you contribute to your world. You just don't operate well without these things.

Only you have responsibility to give these things to yourself. Also for what you do, think, feel and talk about, especially regarding yourself. This is what creates your personal reality. So what do you need right now, what you are not getting? What keeps getting put off or neglected, what are you not getting around to or dealing with? Not sure? Perhaps your unmet need is on your mind right now, so guess what, attend to it right now – take the first step and make a date for the rest. This is how you begin. If you are not sure what you need, listen again to the wisdom of your own heart and find out!

Signs of Unmet Needs

Maybe you are getting the messages, are hearing that you need to rest or take care of yourself, but the bigger picture is not quite resolved and that's holding you back. Don't let it. Give yourself what you need anyway, because if anything is not working in your life right now, it is a direct result of your needs not being met or perhaps your attempt to distract yourself and others from the fact that you actually have needs. For example, do you get disappointed when people don't meet your expectations, let you down or don't behave in the way that you would like them to, or do you sometimes feel unappreciated, unloved and unsupported. If so it means you are not getting what you need.

The issue is always about caring for yourself. Pointing a finger at others just means that you have not fully accepted your pain.

When you are critical and judgmental, or angry and full of resentment, you will have an unmet need lurking around somewhere. Ask yourself where and when this happens. Ask what is working in your life and what isn't. Step up, buy the classier model. Take charge of your life by evaluating what things are and are not working for you and then do something about it – go on, give yourself what you need and reap the rich rewards! The trick is to get what you need and feel totally self-fulfilled and content regardless of what other people do or don't do for you, and to feel the way you want to feel regardless of what you have or have not.

However much you would like others to take care of you, it is ultimately your own responsibility to see that you get the love, care, attention and fun that you need. Giving yourself the right attention builds up your self-esteem and is a signal to the world that you are an important human being.

On those occasions when you do need to ask another for something, ask in a way that can be clearly understood: "I need you to want me; believe me; understand or trust me" actually doesn't tell the listener a thing! You must actually SAY what that looks like:

"I need you to stop checking my mobile phone for messages from other lovers," then I'll know you trust me!

"I need you to bring me flowers on a Friday and tell me how pretty my hair looks, or wolf-whistle when I'm ready to go out for the evening," then I'll know you want me.

Concrete, specific needs, NOT generalities. If I ask you to 'respect' me, you may think you know what I mean, but in fact you probably won't. And no matter how hard you try, I can always accuse you of falling short, because we never agreed on what you would have to do specifically to show me respect. The same of course is true of all generalities from 'loving me' to 'giving me space' to, in the case of children especially, 'being good.' These are just labels.

Being clear and taking simple actions builds self-esteem. If your needs are met, your feelings of worth and empowerment blossom and your relationships improve dramatically. If the other isn't willing, however, to meet or even negotiate your needs, you have a clear signal that the relationship may be part of the problem. Whatever happens, take care of yourself now. Things may not be exactly as you would want them in an ideal world, but take action, look after yourself now. When you look after yourself in this way, the emotions won't get too far out of control in the first place.

Beware of Sabotaging Through Self-Criticism

You also need to ensure you are not causing the emotions, causing the neediness yourself. Stay aware of your self-talk around the whole issue, as this is often where you can sabotage clarity. In other words stop listening to your small self – "I've felt sad/lonely/angry since my partner 'left me' – hark at the disempowerment in those two words!

Then we tell nasty stories about ourselves. For example, in response to the thought: "I feel sad and lonely because my partner left me," the 'negative self' responds: "That's because you let yourself get fat and nagged too much."

The self-criticism continues: "He said as much himself; he was always looking at slimmer women and his mother said that you brow-beat him. Why, even your own family is always saying how bossy you are."

So during vulnerable times, you repeat the critical words of others, past or present. Then you try to ignore or pretend the ensuing tears aren't there; call yourself stupid, weak or neurotic for having them; give yourself a further slagging off and just in case that wasn't enough, label yourself for it and take the blame. Just to be certain, you back it up by a short but very precise character assassination right down to the core of who you are. This type of self-inflicted disempowerment serves up a cocktail of feelings that leaves you full of self-loathing and worthlessness. Yes self-criticism works every bit as well as affirmations, only putting you down rather than building you up – is that your true intent?

I know I've done a great job of keeping myself small and feeling dirty deep inside in my time. Shall I add all the self-defeating behaviours that accompany that? In other words, all the really beneficial things we do to achieve anaesthesia when we decide: 'F-this; time to jump off the mountain.' I thought so. You know the pattern so well. I've seen it so frequently in my work that I often get a chuckle when I reel off this kind of thinking specific to clients. I sum it up so well they think I have read their minds, but I'm no psychic; it's simply that this type of thinking is so common.

Suppression

Suppression is another good one (a common unhelpful response to emotions), i.e., pretending you don't feel and you don't hear. Denial. The thing is, denial is hard work; apparently the body has to produce a drug 200 times more powerful than morphine to repress all that ugly stuff – and you wonder why you are tired!

What's worse is we cannot selectively numb emotions. We can't pick out the fear and the anger and the jealousy and say: nice glass of red for the fear; bag of crisps – all that crunching and swallowing – will be great for the anger; and a yummy bar of chocolate usually washes away the jealousy – and actually, I can pretend I'm giving myself a treat. No. Unfortunately, you can't be that picky. You numb it all out, the good with the bad. Surely it is time to wake up!

"We are the most in debt, obese, addicted and medicated adult cohort in history." Brene Brown

Here's something that always helps me to acceptance:

Grant me the serenity
To accept the things I cannot change,
The courage to change the things I can,
And the wisdom to know the difference

So accept the situation, accept where you are right now, acknowledge and own your feelings in it. A simple hands up will do while taking note of how you say it:

"I feel angry" is quite different to "I am angry." The former allows you to then disassociate from the emotion. You are Mary, Jane, Tom, Dick or Harry, but you are not angry. You are Mary, Jane, Tom, Dick or Harry, and you may at this moment feel angry – excuse me, psychotherapists have to be pedantic; it comes with the territory and it can make all the difference.

If you find yourself sitting back on a barge like the King or Queen of 'De Nile,' you just have to work harder at the becoming-aware-of and getting-to-know-yourself part, ergo, Temple of the Heart: Looking Within. Once you've let go of the emotional charge of it, are back on undulating hills and able to think again, you can give your own process a little scrub up. Ask what you are actually saying to yourself. In our example above ("I've felt sad since my partner 'left me'"), try instead: "I've felt sad lots since we parted." It takes out the victim, claiming more responsibility for you.

When working with couples, I always say it's fifty/fifty: there cannot be a bully without a victim. It doesn't matter if it is literally true or not; blaming is a game where there is no winner, so it's just not a healthy way of looking at it. I know it can feel better when you have someone to blame, but the truth is, if you take away the responsibility you have to yourself, you are simply abdicating an opportunity to move on and bring yourself to another level of process and acceptance.

"I felt angry about his affair, but I am learning to accept that it said more about him than it did about me. Next time, I will follow my gut instinct. I'm now building a life of my own, shaky as it is."

Get the gist? Embrace acceptance and take responsibility for your life. Let go of the emotional charge, take proper action on your true needs moment to moment. This will lead to another level of acceptance from which you can again observe, this time, your self-talk around the event. In your calmer state you can then rewrite the script, which in turn leads towards manifesting what you are truly seeking.

I know first-hand that when something big happens, the initial accepting may just be momentary, but in the end that is all you have, each and every blessed moment. Kinda up to you how you spend them. Make the most of each and every one, so that even in times of pain and grief you can find some calm, some resolve, the ability to detach, see what is really going on and find a peace within. That peace will come from the self-awareness, which builds with daily practice.

A client once told me they worried about something all day long. Really – all day? Well, 6-8 hours, they said. I counted it up, that's 7 hours a day on average, about 50 hours a week or 2,500-3,000 hours a year! Imagine if I were to give you a gift of 3,000 hours a year. What would you do with it? What would you do with it if there were absolutely no limits? What if I waved my magic wand and removed all limitations? Just exactly how would you be living your life in that case? Great thought.

Add up the hours you spend worrying, obsessing, on or off diets, nursing the hangover or feeling stressed, and spend it focusing on the things you are learning right now, on your desires. How amazing would that be? Think of all the stuck energy you'd be releasing. And let's face it: if the only real alternative is to continue to jump off the mountain, which will never lead you to where you want to go. Isn't it time to change course?

A cared-for body, properly directed thoughts, realised and released emotions and a physiological state born of conscious choice is not only your greatest ally in fighting disease and maintaining radiant health and energy, but can also be the platform to living the life of your dreams. So...

Process the emotions, don't let them process you, use e-motion to grow.

Use the self-knowledge you've discovered, practice the techniques, which bring you to the frequency you intend to be. The thing is, if you don't, not only are you missing the opportunity of utilizing e-motions as a vehicle to move forward in your life, but your body ends up processing them for you. If anger can deform a water cell, just think of what holding anger for years and years would do to your body. In fact, they say that the disease of anger is cancer – the deeper the anger, the more virulent the cancer – your diseases and illnesses can tell you more about yourself and your life. Think about it: sinusitis – who's getting up your nose? Bad back – lack of support. Weight gain – protection. Incontinence – emotional overflow; and so on. It's your body's way of attracting your attention and asking you to look at a specific area of your life that is in need of re-energising. Acknowledge your symptoms too. They are just other hints on the road to self-knowledge.

An inner glow develops as you get to know and love yourself: eat the food that nourishes you, take the exercise your body needs and are gentle within your own mind. Nurture a quiet sense of self-respect, a feeling of self-worth. Be grateful and glad that you are you!

Well done!

Time to let go of the past…

Chapter 5

MASTERING THE PAST

The ancients were holistic practitioners. They believed in the healing power of catharsis, and of sleep. Sleep was used not only to heal but as a training tool for neophytes in the temple programme.

You too can use catharsis and sleep to heal your past and to redirect your future.

You are not your past...

The past may have helped make you who you are, but you are not your past.

Ancient Sleep Temples, Catharsis and Holistic Healing

The belief in the healing power of catharsis goes back to the sleep temples of Imhotep, and the word catharsis comes from the Greek katharos, meaning 'to purify.' Sleep temples were well established in the ancient worlds. They were for healing – ancient hospitals if you like – treating a variety of ailments, many psychological in nature. Healing was holistic, dealing with the deep underlying cause of a problem rather than addressing the symptoms. Going deeper and asking those hard questions helps you to take responsibility for your own life, to heal, to grow, to develop personally and spiritually, becoming more of whom you really are, always were, and can be right now.

Ancient healing included metaphor, suggestion, alchemy, dream analysis, and sound and energy work. I have no doubt the ancients were masters, and would have used a combination of methods to heal people of all sorts of problems, both physical and mental.

In the Sleep Temples of Imhotep, where inscriptions on the walls tell of miraculous cures, the sick participated in rituals, were put into trance and told that the priests would 'cast out' bad spirits from the mind and body so that a healing by the gods would take place. Treatment was usually preceded by a cleansing ritual: meditation, fasting or bathing, as well as sacrifices to the patron deity or other spirits. Chanting was used to place the recipient into a trance or hypnotic state, and the ensuing dreams would then be analysed in order to determine treatment. Everything was done to achieve catharsis – in other words, a purification through emotional release.

After their journey to the healing temple, the seekers would write their request on papyrus or lobby someone to speak on their behalf then wait around the peripheries until it was deemed the right moment for them to enter. They would be cleansed and, where necessary, go through a further clearing process, perhaps a fast. You can still see rituals of purification on the temple walls today. After cleansing, the seeker would be anointed. Again, the ancients, with their knowledge of alchemy, would have certainly known which elixirs and essences would induce the correct state of mind. Finally the seeker would be clothed in special robes before entering the actual sanctuary.

Once inside and made comfortable, seekers would have their 'consultation' and if, for instance, a man had glaucoma ('clouds over his eyes'), the priest or priestess would say it represented clouds in the sky blocking clear sight of Ra. To heal it, they would first tell the story of how Ra conquered his enemies and was victorious. The psychological preparation was completed through incantation and ritual to bring on a deep trance-like sleep, during which suggestions would be given to summon dreams from the gods. The ancient Egyptians believed that their culture came directly from the gods themselves and there are plenty of mysteries to support this theory. They believed that the ba, or soul, travelled during sleep and collected the dream, a message from the gods, which the priests and priestesses would interpret to find a cure. Today we call it a message from the subconscious. Freud himself said dreams are the royal road to the subconscious mind. Your subconscious mind can supply you with nightly entertainment in the shape of personalised movies, and you can encourage it by writing out your dreams first thing every morning.

Whatever you wish to call it – the power of suggestion, magic, or intervention of the gods – is up to you. The sleep temples were massively successful and copied through Greek and Roman cultures. Temple sleep was used as a psychotherapeutic tool, and a healing occurred. You can see the similarities to hypnosis today. People then, as now, wanted solutions to their problems; they wanted to lay down their burdens and to be content in their lives.

Not so different to what we want today.

Letting Go - Emotional Cleansing

In psychotherapeutic terms, catharsis means releasing unconscious conflicts. There are many ways of releasing, some helpful, some less so. You have a choice in how to deal with your feelings of frustration, hurt, anger, disappointment, and grief.

Let's say you experience stress over a work-related situation. You could go home and vent on your other half, the kids or the cat; drown your sorrows in a chilled glass of crisp white wine; swallow it down with a large tub of ice cream or trance out in front of the telly – maybe all of the above! Alternatively, you can find release by working out your problems. Working things out will help physically, mentally, emotionally and spiritually, and be much kinder to all concerned, especially you. Using your self-knowledge, be honest and get down to the nitty-gritty, then use the power of catharsis to let it go.

Find release or catharsis in two ways.

You need to let go of the emotional charge of everyday situations as an ongoing way of looking after yourself. I hope that through practices of the preceding chapter that you are already beginning to see you are the master of your emotions, not the other way around. You also need to let go of built-up emotional charges from the past.

Holistic Model: Symptom

Let me explain. Think of the mind as a cup that fills up with stress and the ordinary things that hurt us all. The dregs at the bottom is the stuff from the past, and your everyday stuff tops it up. When the cup becomes full, the feelings begin to overflow in unhelpful ways, or perhaps you experience the onset of a symptom. A symptom is simply the subconscious mind letting you know something needs attention. The subconscious mind doesn't talk to you in your head in quite the same way as the internal nag or the superhero self (negative and positive egos); rather, it talks to you in subtle ways: through the language of the body, through the language of dreams and of the universe (messages from the gods). One way or another you will be sent the same message over and over again until it dawns on you – I need to hear this! If you continue to ignore the messages, the symptom will only get worse. This is most often the stage clients have reached when they walk through a therapist's door. They've become absolutely overwhelmed by the feelings and/or the physical manifestation of those feelings.

Feelings

Let me clarify exactly what I mean by feelings. You could say that emotions are objective, the physical response to something that occurs in your world. Emotions can be measured in physical responses – body language, blood flow, brain activity. Feelings on the other hand are subjective; feelings are the meanings we give to emotions, and how we interpret them. We are not taught much about either one.

We are sent to school to learn how to use our brains, to after school clubs for hobbies and to social events, dancing and so on, to learn to mix with others. However, as far as feelings go, the little we do learn tends to be governed by stereotypical statements such as "boys don't cry" or "girls don't get angry." We simply don't get lessons in dealing with anger, hurt, frustration, jealousy, and the loneliness of not quite connecting with others.

Yet there is no question: feelings can be uncomfortable, not only our feelings, but those of others too. So we learn to push our feelings down, to bottle them up. The trouble is, this can cost us dearly. It takes a lot of energy to keep those feelings down, energy we could use to simply get on with and enjoy life. It's not healthy to keep our feelings locked up, but each time a phrase like "Don't be angry!" or "Get on with it" is used, the way we feel is invalidated and a little part of us begins to doubt ourselves. We begin to think that we must be wrong and those other voices must be right. We still feel what we feel; it just gets easier to store it away somewhere inside. The long-term effects of having our feelings denied is not trusting our feelings, and, eventually, not feeling at all.

Yet despite that, and in a very real sense, those feelings are still with you. Like will always attract like, so if, for example, as a child you went through the same type of upset over and over again, you may still be creating the same situation in your present. These things can be cumulative, and when there is enough of the same type of reactions, an unhealthy pattern is established and disease or illness can result; your wonderful body ends up processing the emotions you are not processing yourself.

So how do you release hurts of the past?

Releasing the Past

You can very easily release hurt from the past and reframe the issue – look at it in a new way. Don't worry, there is no need to do every single hurt in your long-legged life; choose one incident at a time and stick with it; it will have a snowball effect. Work through those that stand out, and the amazing healer called the subconscious mind will sort out the rest.

"There's nothing in the past to worry about. The past has gone; it's left behind its memories and the lessons it taught. But the past has gone; there's nothing in it to concern yourself with. "There's nothing in your future to be conscious about, because the future's not yet; and, when it arrives, it will be the present, a precious gift." William Carr

Talking It Out

A friendly ear also helps. Do whatever gets it off your chest. If you don't have someone close with whom to talk your feelings out, there are plenty of therapists around, including voluntary services. You don't need to do this in isolation; you might be amazed at just how little it takes. For instance, what do you think the average number of therapy sessions is? I was amazed when I found out that the mean number of talking therapy sessions is one! Research shows that many clients feel so much better after one session that they don't need to come back. The issue may not be completely resolved, but the offload helped to the extent that they find themselves in a position to cope. I know from my own experience that the vast majority of clients report a 30-60% improvement after the first session, and often that one is enough.

Writing It Out: Journaling

If you just cannot open up to another person, there are other ways of letting the emotions out. For some of us, writing down thoughts and feelings can be more helpful than conversation. Getting it out through writing relieves the internal stress. So if you find it hard to speak about deep emotions, haven't cried in years, have suffered experiences you are reluctant to discuss, or have no friendly ear to hear you, a session with pen and paper may serve you well.

Daily writing in a journal is something you can do easily to escalate your own healing process. It doesn't have to be a journal; you can write out your deepest thoughts and feelings through stories, letters, and diaries. Lots of my clients have benefited from writing letters, getting even the most deep-seated hurts and angers out, then just burning the paper, letting it go. If it's your style, you can be ritualistic about it. Destroy the paper in three different ways: three is a powerful number, the number of manifestation.

Despite modern technology, the best method is actually writing by hand, as this stimulates your body to produce more natural killer cells, a crucial element in your immune system. Don't worry about the mechanics or grammar; you can always do corrections later if you must. One of my biggest breakthroughs in writing was attending a class where I had to write for six minutes without pause. If I got stuck, I had to write the last word on the page over and over until something else came through. I was amazed at what came out: both deep insights to my hurt and suffering, and a creative flow I had never experienced before. It can work for you too.

If writing doesn't do it for you, there are many other ways. Many people like to let go of physical and emotional tension through movement. Move in any way you wish. Zorba the Greek, mourning his lover, dances it out. You can scream from the mountaintops. Write, talk, dance or sing it out.

All these methods are cathartic and purifying. As you feel the emotions so you can let them go, it may hurt for a moment or two, but it's much better than stagnating with the internalised thoughts and feelings that keep you stuck in the past. Each time you do so, you take another step towards self-knowledge, towards your true self.

Be Honest

Always state YOUR truth as you know it now; don't make it better than it actually is, but don't make it worse, either. Say it as it is. Embellishments or hiding from the truth is still holding onto it, and deludes you into believing it won't hurt as much or that it will go away eventually. Honestly stating your truth as you experience it may even free you from shame. It will certainly clarify your thoughts and feelings. Express it without judgment; judgment may be the very reason you wanted to keep your feelings and thoughts inside in the first place. So let it all out, let it go!

While you are burdened, you simply cannot bloom. So let go and let grow!

Acknowledge problems where they exist and ask yourself honestly if there is an action needed. Facing up to things, accepting what you yourself are responsible for and making amends where appropriate can open the door to what's next.

In my experience, there is then but one thing that can prevent moving on, and that is a lack of forgiveness. Forgiveness is an absolute necessity for psychological wellbeing and health. Here's an example from a client of mine.

Forgiveness

Abbey is a self-confessed pragmatist and atheist, someone who likes 'real things that can be explained with evidence, science and preferably a nice mathematical formula!' In her own words, she has "no time for things like crystal therapy: rocks that can make you feel better...really? And my personal favourite...angel therapy! You might as well offer me pixie therapy and be done with it. I mean, no offense to those who do subscribe to those things, I just don't think that's who I am. I don't see why I shouldn't say so. I do, however, believe in the power of the mind and the brain."

Abbey had fought with weight issues her whole life. I could see there was unresolved conflict holding her back stemming from an awful series of family-related events which resulted in Abbey feeling a huge sense of injustice and unable to even speak with her sister. It seemed there was no way out, and Abbey was understandably very angry. The injustice was so great that when her mother forgave the sister, it just made matters worse. This had been the status quo for two years – and you know what harbouring those sorts of feelings can do. Anyway, I helped Abbey realise that she had to forgive in order to move on. It wasn't easy and took a couple of attempts. Here are her words:

"When in my heart I genuinely had forgiven, really let go of all those bad feelings, a very strange thing happened. Less than four days later, an event occurred which brought about changes that I would not have considered possible. My mum unexpectedly ended up in hospital after an accident. It meant the family had to pull together to help her, my sister and I together. Although some things remain unresolved, I've been able to see the rest of my family without animosity and we have a way forward. It's not the solution I had envisaged; I didn't get to have the big showdown where everyone got to hear of how unjustly I had been treated, but there was a solution. The logical part of my brain says 'coincidence,' but a newer, more open part of my heart says something different. I had to let go before a solution was presented. I had to forgive and move on, and once I had, that blockage, that conflict, was removed and I was able to focus on me. And hey, and I've lost a few pounds already..."

Wonderful story, eh? I love it, and whether you think it is all pixies and coincidences is up to you. I see this on a weekly basis in my work, and as the great man said:

"Coincidence is God's way of remaining anonymous." Albert Einstein

The Energy of Forgiveness

So I believe forgiveness is an absolute necessity for personal and psychological health, a must-do for your wellbeing and growth. None of the above is worth the paper it is written on when you continue to harbour resentment in your heart. To refuse to forgive is to remain a victim imprisoned by the past, held in chains of perpetual anger, resentment, pain and bitter unhappiness, locked in old grief that will never, ever serve you and always be excruciatingly detrimental to your own self. I have seen clients continue to yield to another's control years after the event through their inability to let go of their own self-righteous outrage and revenge. These responses poison their every precious moment. How sad. What a waste. Perhaps you've heard this before, but it bears repeating: Refusing to forgive is like drinking poison and waiting for the other person to die. It simply doesn't work.

Yet forgiveness can be a difficult step to take, and I have witnessed clients' anger when I dare to even use the word 'forgive.' I see it again when I feedback in equal measure the words, facial expressions and tense body contortions that is the legacy of this bitter stuff. Then I say, "OK, so you want to stay like this?" That usually does it: they see themselves reflected in me and realise the hurt they are doing to themselves. The seed has been planted.

Forgiveness is a process, a journey you must make again and again if you are to remain happy. To forgive doesn't benefit those who did you wrong; it benefits YOU. It is one of the most cathartic and empowering things you can do for yourself. In forgiveness, you create a new beginning, let go of hurts from the past and of emotional burdens that were probably never yours in the first place. To not forgive is to remain the victim and to wallow in the repeating mantra of your boring old past and hurt pride. You also have to forgive yourself – in fact, very often the greatest hurt is the hurt you do to yourself, and for sure that is the one you get most angry about.

Forgiveness also takes courage, especially when you think the injustice seems too great, but like most things, the more often you do it, the easier it becomes. It doesn't matter what they have done – if they've said sorry, made amends or been punished – because this is about you, not them. It's about you taking your power – the power to free yourself from the bonds of the past.

Free yourself from the past – forgive!

So let me ask you – is there a situation of yours that has come to mind while reading this? If so, what state do you get into when you think about it? Is that it? Do you want to remain like this? Is that how you choose to live your life? Beware that when anger and hatred have been living in your heart for long enough, you become used to it. It becomes the devil you know, and you may even grow to like your grudges and hatreds. Is that what you want? Wouldn't life be better without those toxic thoughts and feelings? Or aren't you ready to let yourself feel that good?

In many cases, the event is in the past, the person is no longer in your life, and the work of forgiveness is done within and around yourself. In other cases, especially when family is involved, it is in your face on a daily basis, yet the circumstances remain out of your control. Despite this being trickier, you can still work on yourself, and yourself, as you know, is the only thing you can change anyway. Paradoxically, when you do change, it has a positive effect on those around you too, and remember you always have the option of stating your case for the record.

Another client, Jayne, had been in a wrangle with very close family for ten years. The situation was one that quite honestly would piss anyone off. I could see why she found it outrageous. She was in a royal rage. The day I fed it all back to her, I thought she was going to walk out. Luckily, I know how to dodge bullets. She came back.

The first step of Jayne's journey to forgiveness was writing out all the hurts of her childhood. They were the same scenarios, issues and feelings that caused the big falling-out, and she felt lighter with each step. I suggested writing a letter. At first even writing one to be burned later seemed as abhorrent as the situation had festered so badly for such a long time. Ten years during which she had met, married and had two beautiful children with her life partner, all without the love and support of her extended family. All done with heavy heart, and carrying a burden that was never hers in the first place.

Eventually, she wrote the letter, and in this case (much to my surprise), decided to send it. Neither of us expected a response, and indeed none was forthcoming, but from that moment on she was free. No longer a victim she started to enjoy her life and enjoy the family members she did connect with. She attended a big family event with her head held high, introducing her young children to all the family; it was up to them if they wanted to be silly buggers. Her children would know all their family and their roots including 'so-and-so the grumpy git' and 'such-and-such the control freak,' and 'Uncle Whatshisname the family drunk.' The kids would discover and realise these things for themselves. My client would never have to face their questions when they got older; they would know.

When you let go of guilt, you will even free yourself from fear. So are you ready to forgive? Here's what Jayne client did.

She remembered the offences with all their horror and wrote them out. This can be painful, but you have all the tools you need. You can do it. We have to feel to heal, and you cannot forgive what you refuse to remember. So even if it is painful, remember what happened, acknowledge it, then write or talk it out and release the emotional charge. Acknowledge, accept and recover that part of you that was lost, and bring it back into the now. See the person you were or simply imagine that energy coming back to you. Be patient; keeping love, freedom of spirit and peace of mind in your heart.

When Jayne was eventually ready to forgive, she simply stated the intention: I intend to forgive and I release myself and everyone else concerned. Later she used an adaptation of a forgiveness technique I was given by Helen Belot, who taught me Sekhem (the communication system and energy used by the ancient Egyptian priesthood). Helen was the first person to drive home to me the importance of forgiveness. She said that when you can forgive the one that has hurt you most, then you truly have arrived. During six years of divorce madness and repeated hurts, I remember thinking, I'll never get there, never. However, my then-husband is my daughter's father, and I could not escape him in this life. I continued to do all the work I taught others, over and over and over again. Yet I doubted I could achieve that which I had convinced others to do. That particular journey of forgiveness was a long and arduous one, laced with new hurts along the way, but I arrived; I got there, and as with all of these things, the prize is greater than you ever imagine.

I believe forgiveness is an initiation to the self, a rite of passage, a freedom. As you take the steps, you may realise that which was indeed your own responsibility, something you had hidden from yourself before, but what we hide is our potential, so forgive yourself, set yourself free and use the energy for a greater good. Decide if the circumstances merit making amends, and if so, then that is what you must do. Repair the damage as best you can. Step by step, move to the compassionate position of wishing well to the person who hurt you. At that point, you will know you have reached the end of your journey and you'll know the trip was worthwhile. Be kind and gentle with yourself along the way; take it in small steps, one foot in front of the other.

Taking time out to acknowledge your feelings and learning new tools is simply a way of developing your self-esteem. As you do this work, take care of your inner dialogue: remember everything from the preceding pages and adapt it to the new you. You will change, you will heal; there is nothing surer. Please don't spoil it by forgetting to update the recording you play in your head! There may be times when you believe you are back in the same old place again, but you are not. You have learned that lesson – remember it! You already know what to do. Do it again and again and again!

Remember, improvement is made in just ONE day:

I forgive myself.

I forgive the past.

I let go.

I release.

I welcome the amazing present that is NOW!

Finding the Temple

Once you've let go of the past, you can focus on the present, a precious gift. How are you treating this present? Are you living the moments that expand you into the greatest and grandest you? Or are you so caught up in the humdrum of your daily do that you are missing what is under your nose, never mind realising those deeper truths that reveal your life's purpose. For those kinds of answers, you need to step back, to draw a line, to retreat to the temple.

Retreat from the humdrum to stillness, to nature, perhaps to connect with like-minded souls, valid ways of hearing your true self and a powerful method of catharsis and growth. Time, space, breath, just for you!

When we begin our journeys, spiritual tours and relaxation retreats, the first step is to relax, to let go of the everyday churn. We tell our stories and get to know ourselves again. In that sharing we can begin to recognise the pieces that have been side stepped or overlooked and realise how to treat our selves henceforth. We learn to re-treat. You and I have done the same thing as we've journeyed through this book: relaxing; building self-esteem; mastering body, mind and emotions; letting go of the past and now embracing the quest to find a quiet stillness within that allows us to find the true essence of ourselves. In everyday life, we are so busy that to fully come back to ourselves, we need that extra distance. It doesn't have to be a life-changing spiritual tour to Egypt or even a weekend away in the hills, just some time for YOU, a momentary pause that is full of intention.

Many of us are just do-ers. I sometimes feel mechanical, I work so hard. However, I learned the art of escape during my daughter's growing up years, years of endless chores and work. I had to. I'd cajole or bribe someone into babysitting, so when it all got too much, I'd leave Friday after work and drive to a place that became an anchor for peace for me. Sometimes I'd share a curry with friends, others I would eat alone, take a walk, then check into to a cosy bed and breakfast and fall asleep early, zzzz! Next morning I'd see the sea. I missed it deeply, living inland and having been brought up on the coast. If my dog wasn't with me, I'd already be missing him, that same fellow I had so resented walking just the morning before. Back to a warm, fluffy bath. No laptop or perpetual mobile back then. Bliss. Home-cooked Scottish breakfast and no washing up! A slow meander home, and in less than twenty-four hours and for the price of petrol and a bed, I felt like I'd had a week off.

There will be something similar you can do. Long or short, learn to make retreat a permanent part of your life. One of the most powerful tools at your disposal, a retreat available on a daily basis, not to mention the best way to chill out ever is Yoga Nidra.

Yoga Nidra

A blissful relaxation for health, healing and deep wellbeing

Yoga Nidra is a powerful technique in which you learn to relax consciously. The direct translation is 'yogic sleep,' but actually it is the body that sleeps while you, remain alert. You lie in absolute stillness as the instructor guides you into a deeply relaxing state from which you will emerge feeling as if you have slept for a month.

Yoga Nidra is a systematic method of inducing complete physical, mental and emotional relaxation. It also has a fine and ancient lineage. Some say that when Atlantis fell, the priests scattered around the world and became the rishis of ancient India as well as the priests of ancient Egypt. Both certainly used the healing power of sleep.

Yoga Nidra will enhance your health, healing and deep wellbeing. It is also a totally satisfying retreat, as my students will absolutely attest to. Yoga Nidra is designed in such a way to guide you quickly into theta consciousness where healing occurs along with a deep sense of relaxation. While in this state you can give yourself, your subconscious mind, and the cosmos, a message of intent. In Yoga Nidra, that message is called the sankalpa, a Sanskrit word which can be translated as "resolution" or "resolve." That resolve will enable you to take the small steps toward creating the frequency you aspire to, put your plan to the cosmos.

It worked for me. During Yoga Nidra teacher training, my sankalpa was: 'I take my time.' What changed was my attitude. I don't know that I actually slowed down, but for the first time in many years I felt I had time, and I have continued to take time for myself, my family and friends, which was what I had been missing. After three or four months practice I had changed something that had been annoying me for a long time. It wasn't difficult. I didn't reschedule or change anything in three-dimensional reality; I just told myself every day, "I take my time," and the quality of my time, felt completely different. So if you want time, tell yourself you take time. If you have struggled with any of the steps in the Resources and

Recordings, use your sankalpa now to rectify that.

For example: "I meditate daily with ease."

Or: "Every day I am getting stronger and fitter."

Taking these small steps and continuously making adjustments will keep you on course. You'll be in good company: Goethe used inspirations and intuitions from the state of Yoga Nidra to solve problems arising in his work. Einstein accelerated his awareness to the speed of light in the famous thought experiments, which led to the theory of relativity. Napoleon would practice for twenty minutes at the height of battle! You too can use it to reach your goals and aspirations, or to simply get back in tune with natural balance and counteract daily stress.

Yoga Nidra is a retreat in your own home with all the ingredients of the ancient sleep temples for only twenty minutes of your time. Such retreat helps reinforce the clarity needed to let the cosmos know your intentions so it can bring you the people, places and experiences to help you on your way. Start with what you know you can change – yourself. Work on the ingredients that will construct the 'you' that you intend to be, step by step through the sankalpa.

Now you are ready to master your destiny.

Chapter 6

MASTERING DESTINY

The ancient Egyptians believed in magick, they believed that they could master their destiny even beyond this life. Indeed, they believed that the gods and goddesses GAVE them the key of life.

You too have the key to mastering your destiny.

You are not your future

Now that you are rocking your body, mind and emotions, have soared above the lessons of the past, and achieved a new level of self-awareness, I guess it's time to talk destiny. You are not your future, but you do have the key to mastering your destiny, so let's discuss the messages you project on to that amazing tool, the subconscious mind, indeed to the cosmos itself.

Since writing this book, it has become strongly grounded in my everyday awareness that the subconscious mind and the cosmos are exactly the same thing. There's nothing quite like writing a transformational book to force you to look the process of manifestation right in the eye, and of course the only measure is your own life. So I asked: what's the best method of communicating with this cosmic consciousness in order to live on purpose and fulfil your destiny?

Manifestation - how do we do it?

One of my earliest gurus said there were four rules of manifestation: desire, imagination, will and expectation.

Desire – yes, definitely, whether conscious or otherwise. Imagination - certainly that too. Imagination is the melting pot, the witch's cauldron, the crucible. However I'm less sure about the other two rules: expectation and will. Expectation would need a bit more interpretation for me, I wonder if it limits the possibility of something even better.

The use of will is something I have dumped in the anal department; it just seems anti-flowing to me, too much trying involved. Besides, using will power is a dangerous game for the addicts amongst us. Now if you swap will for action, I might agree. There are certainly times when you need to take action, times when no amount of willing, expecting, desiring, or acting 'as if' will do it. Let me give you an example.

More Spiritual than Practical

I fancied owning a sports car, so I put the glossy brochure on my desk and placed a crystal on top of it. I looked at it every day while sending it Sekhem. I even imagined sitting in it, smelling the new leather, feeling the pulsating engine and hearing it purr alongside Meat Loaf's 'Like a Bat out of Hell.' Oh yes, that felt good.

Maybe three years later, bored of dusting it, my then-husband said to me, "Can you not afford your car yet, Vicki?" I thought about it. "I suppose I could." "Well, you will actually have to go out and buy it!" he replied. It was true; I had somehow thought it would just turn up on the doorstep with a pink bow around the bonnet. Oops, I had forgotten the action step!

So you see, it's not enough to really want something, not enough to visualise it over and over again: you have to match your dreams with actions, and all of the above needs to be in alignment with the highest purpose.

I pretty much thought that was it. I wrote out my list of outcomes and when I found them six months later was pleasantly surprised that I was able to tick most of them off. One noticeable failure however, was 'a happy and loving family.' I couldn't understand. This was the thing I desired most and worked hardest at; I willed it and imagined it all the time. I practiced gratitude for what we did have every day. Yet it took ten years.

The universe eventually gave me the happy and loving family I'd asked for, but it was not the family I had had, nor even imagined having when I asked. I sometimes wondered what would have happened if I didn't put that intention out there. Did I initiate the dissolution of my marriage? Was I asking for something that could never be true within that particular situation? I didn't understand why my other wishes came true and not that one. Realisation came once I had that happy family – an unconventional, but nevertheless happy family. I looked back at how hard I'd tried, how much energy I'd given. I had taken all the right steps, said all the right words, I'd even performed the rituals. However, I was stuck; in fact, it seemed the more I tampered with it, the worse it became – that was because it was simply not my path. There were many other lessons to learn before my true path became clear.

What I found even more puzzling was that there were many other times when manifestation was as easy as "abracadabra." Indeed, magick often occurred when I was just mucking around.

Unintentional Affirmations

My funniest experience of manifestation while mucking around was while teaching affirmations. The response to: "I, Vicki, now have lots and lots of money, a six-pack and a gorgeous toy boy" was so good that I kept it going. This entailed lots of writing and repeating. I'm not sure if it was a subconscious desire, but I was certainly 'excited,' in 'peak state,' and having lots of fun as I repeated it over and over while doing the 'Curly the Cougar' strut and imagining toy boys chasing me down the street. It was only when I went back to do the class a year later that I realised it had actually come true. I have no idea if it was coincidental, or because I had reached the age of the cougar: attractive: empowered, self-confident, and independent, but, I was pleasantly surprised when I realised I had my six-pack back, was earning much more than the year before and indeed had begun what turned out to be a wonderful relationship with a much younger man – all done in fun.

Too much detail

I've had the reverse happen too due to having far too much detail on my ideal partner list. If only I'd worked a little more on who I needed to be and stated simply: 'my ideal partner' and trusted the universe to deliver, things would have been much easier. Instead, I made a list, a very long list, but unfortunately I had missed out a few key ingredients. Oh well, we live and learn.

So it seems to me that at times manifestation stays tantalisingly beyond reach no matter whose theory you follow, while at other times your greatest desire just pops in seemingly uncalled for. Times when it seems you can do no wrong. In fact, it is often when you are feeling nonchalant and humorous that the universe seems to obey every click of your fingers.

However, whether intentionally or otherwise, you do have to declare yourself: you need to commit.

I will always remember what Erika called her "eureka moment."

"After sorting out some of the issues that I felt were dragging me down or holding me back in life, it was time to tackle one of the main problems that had been niggling me since my teenage years – my inability to select a good partner. In my twenties I'd brushed it off as not wanting to settle down (thinking back, I was possibly kidding myself even with that statement) but when I reached thirty this started to get me down – why did I choose these losers? I actually cringe when I think of some past relationships – what was I thinking?"

During one session, Vicki and I began discussing 'wish lists' and she asked me what was on my list when it came to my ideal partner – I realized I couldn't answer her, I didn't have a clear list of the qualities required by my ideal partner – either written on paper or simply stored in my mind. The only thing I could think of was, pathetically, that they 'fancied me.'

Reflecting back now, I can see that this started in my early teens. I was an awkward, shy teenager, I never seemed to fit in with the cool crowd of girls and none of the boys ever asked me out. Then on a school trip to Newcastle, I ended up being kissed by one of the boys. Until that moment, I'd never even considered him as attractive…then when he showed a slight interest in me, it was almost as if I was proving to the rest of the group 'Look – he finds me attractive, I'm normal!

I regarded my status within the female popularity ranks as pretty low. I felt I was just marginally above the 'weird' kids that didn't talk to anyone. Therefore, it kind of made sense that I should be grateful that another being should find me attractive and that my attraction to them naturally came second; I had been brought up with a 'not to think above yourself' and 'be grateful for small things' mentality. So in terms of a 'list,' them fancying me was the only requirement, I should feel lucky that somebody does.

So this started a chain of terrible relationships – guys who drank, used drugs, ones with extensive baggage from past relationships, lads who had dead end jobs, no jobs, one guy who beat me up (difficult one to break, as usually when he was begging forgiveness for his actions, his adoration for me increased), and sadly also a few men who were married/in relationships. The prize here of course was the fact that plain old me – low on the popularity rank – had managed to steal a partner from somebody far higher up the chain, so obviously I was the winner there. But they all fancied me at the start of the relationship, and that's all I was asking for wasn't it?

My poor parents…

Vicki set me the task of rewriting my wish list and from there on things started to change – I started to value myself, realized that I was allowed to ask for better things and I questioned myself as to what I wanted; I wanted children, I wanted a man who had good values, I wanted stability, I wanted somebody to fit in with my family.

Don't get me wrong – I took a few wrong turns after that, but I then managed to identify problems quickly and deal with them. If I went on a date with somebody then found they didn't match the requirements of my list, I didn't sleep with them, I didn't take them to my works night out or cousins 21st or even sign off Christmas cards with their name (why did I do this anyway? Such was my desire to be seen as part of a couple, obviously). I just ended it there and continued in my quest to find Mr. Right who matched my list, and eventually I found him – honest, funny, great father to our children, adored by my own family, and if I squint my eyes when he is wearing sunglasses, he does look a bit like Kelly Jones from the Stereophonics even if that's just in my own head."

Thanks for sharing that Erika – and as you and I know, in your head is the only place where it matters!

Erika found her happy ever after and is now helping others realise that they too are more, helping them to stop, take a moment to think and ask themselves: "What do I really want?"

Asking the question is crucial. At one stage I was scared of stating what I desired, because I was frightened of manifesting yet another big mistake. Then I learned to ask bigger questions. I continued to check out my needs by looking into my heart on a daily basis, but once I accepted I wasn't totally alone in the creation process, that there was a bigger power at work, I started asking questions outside myself. "Who do I need to be to attract the perfect partner, job, house, mind set and experiences into my life?" "What would be good for me right now?" "What am I grateful for right now?" When I am confused, I ask: "What is the gift in this situation?" I also ask, "What is my gift to share right now?" And "What is my gift to the world?" These types of statements are openers; they create a state of openness that attracts all of the right things toward you in perfect divine right timing.

I am sure you have discovered on the road to self-mastery that your greatest ally is taking pause, finding a stillness within which gives the awareness that is key. The stillness is also a shift in state, which, however short, can be looked at as showing up. The trick is to show up enough to demonstrate that you are asking for and ready to receive that change. The universe hears you best when you step back and have the receiver button switched ON! Your future can be changed; it is your creation. However, a note of warning here.

These techniques are based on ancient practices and they do work, so be careful what you ask! Learn from the process itself. Think about what you really want or just ask for 'something better' or 'the perfect solution.' Also ask for recognition that the process is working; wonderful assurances will be given to you at this level of awareness, and 'coincidences' or synchronicities will multiply. Times when things seem so wrong have a way of turning out perfectly in ways you just couldn't have guessed if you simply ask then let it go. But do ask because:

"Until one is committed, there is hesitancy, the chance to draw back. Concerning all acts of initiative (and creation), there is one elementary truth that ignorance of which kills countless ideas and splendid plans: that the moment one definitely commits oneself, then Providence moves too. All sorts of things occur to help one that would never otherwise have occurred. A whole stream of events issues from the decision, raising in one's favour all manner of unforeseen incidents and meetings and material assistance, which no man could have dreamed would have come his way. Whatever you can do, or dream you can do, begin it. Boldness has genius, power and magic in it! Begin it now." Goethe, 'Commitment'

Commitment switches the receiver button on, puts you into a stream of energy and a wave of coincidences that will pick you up and take you where you need to go.

However, commitment is nothing without congruence. Indeed, one without the other is exactly when the ride can become very bumpy.

Realise what is real and what is role.

Back in the days when I energised crystals over shiny car brochures, a Mercedes Benz and a Sekhem teacher weren't things that you connected.

Footballer's wife yes, healer, no. I have since learned that both the blonde in the sports car and the Sekhem teacher dressed in purple were roles I played and indeed enjoyed. However, back then I judged it to mean I was a phony, a cheat, a charlatan. I read an article saying it was impossible to focus on both money and spirituality. Yet my insight told me I could 'have it all,' and for years I felt strongly that part of my 'service contract' was to help others realise that they too could have it all. I so desperately didn't want to be the skint saint that, instead of trusting my intuition, I made an agreement with the 'invisible forces that be' to continue going where work led me so long as I was looked after, that the means would come. It did.

I had in fact stumbled on the formula but misunderstood why it had worked. It worked because of who I was being. Those things I'd felt I was being 'forced' to learn were in fact already within me, and certain energies, people and places drew it out. I saw the same in my students.

I have it all within me and so do you. The whole point is to share your special and unique gift. Humankind is endogenous – we embrace it all. To fulfil our purpose and to flourish, we simply have to release it; in the same way as flowers have to release their seeds, we have to share our gift.

The universe has always been regarded as the source of all life. Matter, which is found within the universe is everywhere, including within us. The ancient Egyptians believed that our souls were stars and that once we died, we would simply return home to shine down upon the living, to guide them in their lives. We embrace all of that within the essence that we are here to seed. The gift of light we are here to share. The ancient Egyptians drew it all over the temple walls, gave us clues everywhere – the gods and goddesses gave us the key of life – use it!

So the incongruence within me had been the lie I told myself: that if my story had a 'happy ever after,' I was OK, but if my marriage failed there was no good in me. This misbelief made me hang on when I needed to let go. The truth is that I was always a spiritual, intuitive woman. The darkness wasn't my past but my present: I was deeply unhappy in my marriage.

Extraordinarily, the part I had hidden, had felt was my incompetency, was the area of my potential and growth. The realisation that the phony part hadn't been ME or my spiritual gifts dawned on me slowly over the ensuing years as I watched others work through their false pride and their shame, I heard how their sexuality and projections could tie them in knots. It was my experiences as much as my training that helped set them free from these things and in return their stories helped me realise that it is not only OK but, imperative that we show up as our true selves, the good, the bad, and the ugly. If we don't, we will never get beyond the shame to our deeper truth.

So now, living in the fire of transformation, at last I have stepped out of self-judgment, into rigorous self-honesty. I have stopped worrying about how I might be perceived, and thus have enabled myself to write and share my journey with you.

In your journey to self-knowledge, I'm sure you'll discover where you have fibbed to yourself too. It's OK, you are wiser now, you can move on, to do that – forgive yourself.

I sat with a client yesterday who felt that everything was just 'wrong' in her life for no apparent reason. Her upbringing was such that she was 'trained' to put up with the unacceptable and selfish behaviour of the man she married. Finally, the veil lifted and she got away, but now in what could be a golden opportunity, nothing seems to be sitting or fitting. So controlled for so long, she was still doing it to herself. What had gone on in that long marriage gave her the material to beat up on herself – arghhh! This is what we can do to ourselves. She was shocked at my suggestion to forgive herself and it was hard for her to stay still enough to recognise that was indeed what she had to do – and of course to stop the fibs. Accept that is what happened and move on.

I am sure you have also recognised many layers and facets of yourself:

"All the world's a stage, and all the men and women merely players. They have their exits and their entrances, and one man in his time plays many parts." Shakespeare

Own it, enjoy it. I laugh as I think of some of the parts I have played. It helps self-acceptance to own your ego in this way. Laying bare your "small self," your ego roles, can of course leave you feeling vulnerable, but humour helps.

Who am I? - starring Pedro and the Page Three Girl

While I was teaching Sekhem in Orkney one year, a member of our group, Ian, said on a couple of occasions:

"Down Pedro, down!" We had to ask, "Who on Earth is Pedro?" "My ego," he replied. He was using the psychological trick of dissociation. Recognising that trait within ourselves, we giggled as we named our small selves. Humour can enable you to recognise when you are in ego, and the more you do so, the more easily you can jump back into true self.

I hesitate to concede that true self is only the spiritual self, as for me true self is made up of many parts and you should feel free to accept those parts so long as they are not holding you back. True self can have surprising and seemingly incongruous elements, like a saint who loves good beer. It's OK to value the disparities so long as they are authentic and healthy. Our parts make us more, not less, and anyway, meditation will take you beyond them, beyond the roles you play in life: mother, father, lover, employee, boss, daughter, son, or friend. What do these things really mean, anyway? Mother, for instance, is so often taken to mean general dogsbody. Roles are too concerned with doing and not concerned enough with being. They won't last forever, and at a deep level you live in fear of losing your part to play, your role. However, when you are in touch with the wisdom within, the self that lies beyond the physical, beyond space and time, you can realise for yourself who you truly are and your connection to all things. Then it is easy to embrace all of your facets and to find self-love in those aspects of yourself that you previously felt ashamed of. Realise they have served their purpose and can be released. You can accept the role you are playing for what it is. Enjoy it: just don't let it be king.

To be in full congruence, to be authentic and to connect with that true self means letting go of false pride, letting go of perfectionism and walking hand in hand with your fear.

False pride is just another way of hanging onto ego or role, of believing that you are your role. Trying to be perfect is a high road to nowhere, like waiting for the perfect moment to do things. The thing is, perfection may never arrive, so don't bother with that. Do it as you are. Just do it. Do something you've always wanted to do, and do it just the way you are. Buy another dress if the old one is too tight now, decorate your messy room with candle light. Take a deep breath, go to the personnel department and tell them what your boss is doing. Do it, warts and worries included, and make the intention clear: my soul is dancing, having fun and refusing to be treated like this!

If you still don't feel ready to step into all that you are, ask yourself: Are you just plain scared?

"Our deepest fear is not that we are inadequate. Our deepest fear is that we are powerful beyond measure. It is our light, not our darkness that most frightens us. We ask ourselves, Who am I to be brilliant, gorgeous, talented, fabulous? Actually, who are you not to be? You are a child of God. Your playing small does not serve the world. There is nothing enlightened about shrinking so that other people won't feel insecure around you. We are all meant to shine, as children do. We were born to make manifest the glory of God that is within us. It's not just in some of us; it's in everyone. And as we let our own light shine, we unconsciously give other people permission to do the same. As we are liberated from our own fear, our presence automatically liberates others."
Marianne Williamson

Recognise that? Well, embrace the fear; use its energy to propel you forward towards the life of your dreams and STOP playing small! You are not being all that you can be when you limit yourself with your own judgment, so step up and allow the energy of who you really are to power that wave of commitment!

If it still doesn't feel right, if there's something still niggling deep inside, ask yourself this: Do you feel worthy of being all that you can be?

The most common reason for still not reaching out for this amazing life, for not taking what is rightfully yours yet what was miraculously designed for you, is feeling unworthy. Yet that's tantamount to walking through a field of beautifully ripened strawberries and not partaking of the fruit. Perhaps you believe that the best fruit is not for you. That's OK; if you have come this far and still don't feel good enough to take the strawberry when you are offered it, you are at the point where you will just have to pretend. When clients call on me for, say, confidence building, I sometimes ask: "Was there ever a time when you felt that confident?" If they have honestly never had such an experience, we look for someone they can model. We talk about how that confident person would speak, look, hold themselves, breathe and so on. Then I guide them in creating the same thing in their mind – their subconscious mind, of course.

Remember that amazing tool that doesn't know the difference between imagination and reality. Hears everything you say, yet deletes all negatives, is hugely visual, prefers symbols and metaphors to words. Stays in constant communication with you, is fantastically obedient, has a great sense of humour and functions better with highly potent, top quality cocktails. Use that.

Then imagine you are plucking and tasting that fruit, glorying in its sweetness, savouring that delicious lemon or that sun-ripened berry, mmmmm, sweet and juicy. Yes, taste that wonderfully sweet strawberry or whatever your favourite fruit is. Eventually the energetic wave YOU create by imagining yourself tasting that favourite fruit will pull you towards plucking and tasting. In other words, play that movie of yours often enough and your amazing body-mind will supply the physiology to convince you to bring it into manifestation. Do it in your imagination, practice, practice, practice, and before you know it you'll be doing it in your life!

This is simply creating the peak state for success. Your peak state is the energy wave within you and thus the energy wave you emit to the universe, the frequency you are broadcasting. This is a key piece, as it doesn't matter what you do – you won't attract what you need if you are not in the right state to receive it. Remember, like attracts like. So being in the right state is not something for once a week on a Sunday morning, or even for half an hour every morning; you need to be constantly aware of and constantly adjusting your state. You do that by being conscious of how you are breathing, hydrating and moving. By mastering your emotions – your chemical factory. Doing what is needed to calibrate your brain, programming it well. Living authentically, imagining well and measuring it against your true intention. Then the only piece of the puzzle that is left is...

Reminders

Make your life a ritual act or set reminders. I use my phone alarm, hold weekly check-in meetings with myself, and take regular getaways to make sure I remember. Seriously, my phone bleeps at regular intervals throughout the day to remind me to wake up, to check in with myself, ask myself if I am in peak state. Do I need to stretch, drink, move? Have I buried a piece of myself today?

I love daily rituals and reminders, having woke up with a shock twice in my life after twelve-year sleeps: heroin, then marriage. The latter was the scariest in that I was leading a 'normal' life, training as a psychotherapist, taking steps on my spiritual path, and therefore I had the awareness to know deep inside that something was wrong. I didn't take action on that insight and found myself twelve years later with a massive cosmic slap around the face. There was a spiritual path for me to travel, one that I had asked for and fully intended, yet I was resisting it like crazy because it meant letting go of what I had decided was my everyday anchor, a self-imposed anchor that prevented me sailing with the wind. So now I always remember the words:

"And then one day you find ten years have got behind you
No one told you when to run, you missed the starting gun."
Pink Floyd

How could I have been so asleep? I love the paradox: asleep, yet not asleep; not asleep, yet not awake. We use it in hypnosis to help induce trance. In life, you could be awake, yet not awake, not awake yet not asleep. It's OK to be in trance, so long as it's one of your choosing. The sad thing is when you do not know it. So there is no shame in setting the alarm. Do whatever it takes.

After tours, resting and taking time for me, in Egypt and Turkey, every time the Mullah calls I take the opportunity to change state. At home in Scotland, the animals let me know. I take fresh air, stop, stretch, dance, or meditate – all valid state-changers: a re-treat can be as short as that.

What could your cue be to stop allowing the outside to distract and bewitch? To remind you to continuously check if what you are saying and doing is actually getting you the results you desire. Are you morphing into the 'you' of your dreams and aspirations? If not, shake off the shackles and step up! You committed to mastery of the body, mind, emotions, and past so you are on the road; there's no turning back; just by reading this you are making a commitment to change, so you may as well take hold of the reins.

In life you are either master or slave. What do you choose? Master the inner universe of your thoughts and feelings, attitudes and actions – don't leave it too late to realise what lies within and how valuable it is.

Like the seekers of the past, you may have to ask for a healing or an insight where required: i.e., get professional help. The fact is, we therapists are simply looking behind your words, drawing out your intention, discovering what you want instead, getting you to state it, and then helping you discover the tools to get there. You already have all the ingredients, all the tools you need right now. Ask the question, you may just get the answer. Remember life keeps changing, change the vision to match – taking the small steps and continuously making the necessary adjustments that keep you on course is what counts.

I know if I take my time, I get the quality of connections my soul yearns for. In the same way, if I exercise, I feel strong and focused. When I feel contented in this way, my life rolls with ease and I attract the people and experiences that make my life soar. You know what makes you feel good too. At this level of awareness, 'coincidences' or synchronicities will multiply. Times when things seem so wrong have a way of turning out perfectly in ways you just couldn't have guessed, if you simply ask, then let it go. I know that you know exactly what makes you feel good too. So go there, be that.

Think about it like this:

"Most people believe that if they 'have' a thing (more time, money, love – whatever) then they can finally 'do' a thing (write a book, take up a hobby, go on vacation, buy a home, undertake a relationship), which will enable them to 'be' a thing (happy, peaceful, content, or in love). In actuality, they are reversing the Be-Do-Have paradigm. In the Universe as it really is (as opposed to how you think it is), 'havingness' does not produce 'beingness', but the other way around. First you 'be' the thing called 'happy' (or 'knowing' or 'wise,' or 'compassionate', or whatever) then you start 'doing' things from this place of beingness – and soon you discover that what you are doing winds up bringing you the things you've always wanted to 'have'."

"The way to set this creative process (and that's what this is ... the process of creation) into motion is to look at what it is you want to 'have', ask yourself what you think you would 'be' if you 'had' that, then go right straight to being."

"In this way you reverse the way you've been using the Be-Do-Have paradigm – in actuality, set it right and work with, rather than against,

the creative power of the universe."

"Here is a short way of stating this principle: "In life, you do not have to do anything. It is all a question of what you are being."
Neale Donald Walsch, Conversations With God

So it's a decision; you don't actually need anything to be, for example, happy. It's not something that comes from outside; it comes from inside, and when you radiate a happy energy you'll be amazed what it attracts into your life. It's about the state you are choosing for yourself moment to moment.

Stated most simply: 'Don't worry, be happy.'

Decide now, be happy, and watch magic enter your life. You have all the tools you need right now. The real you is already there, perfect and intact. So the most important thing is to BE real and BE happy.

Be Real

The first time I went to Egypt, I connected with Lucy, now a very dear friend. Early in the trip sitting around the pool, we discovered that not only had we both lived in London in the 70s, but knew many people and places in common. Between Lucy and Alex, a young actor with a glamorous celeb girlfriend, I found myself starting to speak for the first time in years about my life as a model and aspiring young actress. I couldn't stop; it felt so good to be heard by ears that bore no judgement.

I'd kept quiet about my past for years, ever since my confession of having been a nude model silenced a lunch of Deeside housewives during the terrifying early days in backwoods suburbia. Not because I'd 'exposed' myself, but because I had done so to the wrong people at the wrong time. More importantly, I had yet to integrate those aspects within myself and was miles from coming to realise or accept the effect that my extrovert sexuality could have on others.

Of course, as soon as I stopped playing small and started being me, I attracted the fabulous friends I have to this day, and ever since that trip to Egypt I became more authentic, more me, more real, and that really was fantastically empowering. My relationship with the group, and with Simon Treselyan, our teacher and facilitator, equalled my spiritual experiences. Indeed, Simon, our guide, Amr and Egypt was the catalyst that set me off touring Scottish sacred sites, like Callanish, which blossomed into facilitating my own retreats, which has been one of the most exciting and satisfying parts of my life. More importantly though, becoming real set me free.

Yet this opening, this vulnerability at the closing of my pages leaves me as a child blushing at my own audacity in the writing. But I don't write because I have the answers; I write because I have a story to tell, part of which is that I love myself as I am now at this exact place on my journey and somehow have achieved something I wish to share. Uncomfortable things still happen, but I make far less of a drama of them. I no longer hide, I keep asking the questions and live every day in gratitude for my journey and for knowing that the answers will come.

I hope you too feel more of a child, willing to ask those questions, "What if?" "What next?" I hope this book has helped you discover a more childlike quality, the road to your true self. When you begin to love yourself by giving yourself what you need each moment and are brave enough to acknowledge and accept, the rest will come. Being authentic necessitates being vulnerable, risking that you are enough, and it is within those risks that you discover the greatest joys.

If you're not real, if there's incongruence within you, well, then you need to do the work. The work will happen whether you like it or not. So be honest. Keep simple practices you can do every single day and you'll get there.

For me, seeking enlightenment while clinging onto a marriage less than joyous was deeply incongruent. Yet interestingly, it was during that time that the messages, dreams and kaleidoscopic visions – experiences I have come to refer to as spontaneous initiations – came thick and fast, just like they had when I needed to see a path away from drugs. They were better than any sci-fi movie I've ever watched. I don't profess to understand it, I just know that I asked for a way out and the universe did everything to let me know how, to wake me up.

Now I trust my own experiences, my own intuition and listen to my heart. I certainly know there are many states of mind and a variety of realities. I encourage you to explore what that might mean for you. Be brave enough to explore other states, new ways of thinking. Dare to see through the illusion while staying grounded, staying in the present and keeping the secret connection that lies within. Make small changes to the things you say and do. Be brave enough to sing like Dereck, to write the letter like Jayne, and to forgive, as Abbey did. For them the piece of the puzzle that was in the way, the very part that was hardest to face, was the way to freedom and truth. Be brave enough to let go.

Embrace Uncertainty

To realise there is most definitely more, to feel, hold and experience that, is magical. All at once you understand that uncertainty is a wonderful and exciting place. Uncertainty touches every part of your existence; is part of your every living moment – embrace it!

I understand living with uncertainty is terrifying. It is even more so for the addicts amongst us. Trying to hold onto a marriage of pain that was actually over before it began, was all about trying to gain certainty in my post-cold-turkey terror. It was a hard lesson, but one for which I am eternally grateful. Realising I wasn't in control, that there was a bigger picture, one I that occasionally got glimpses of, enabled me to live and dance in the uncertainty of life. That ability has brought me more joy than I had ever previously known. It taught me to enter the mystery consciously and intentionally, to enjoy witnessing the how – the amazing way all this works, and discovering the more.

Living in the mystery is an intentional step, a commitment and an initiation. The hawk flies elegantly because he rides the wind, he knows where he is going, he has a destination in mind but he doesn't try to control the wind, he rides the wind. So, amazing being, choose what you REALLY want, what you truly desire, imagine it already being true. Commit to it. Use the power of thought and the power of intention to BE who you intend to be – live in that state and use your subconscious mind to create your vision of your future.

Nothing exists that did not first exist as pure thought; the laws of physics have proven this: thoughts move outward in patterns, like waves from a radio. Most of us are not aware of it, never having been taught, but your mind knows what to do. It's just that for years you haven't been paying proper attention, but believe me, this is how you manifest your experience: through your choices, belief systems, intentions, and fears – conscious or otherwise! That's why we continually need those reminders to stay awake and aware. Your future can be changed, guided by the pictures you make and the thoughts you think; therefore, your intention is crucial because of the energy it is constantly pulling toward you.

In many ways, this book is designed to convince you of just how amazing you are and to provide steps that will constantly remind you to stay awake to that, as well as sharing the 'antidotes' to the common stumbling blocks to living a quality life. With the right mind-set, vehicle and intention, you start living the dream, walking your talk and dancing in the flames of transformation. Then you can caress the uncertainty, the joy of discovery, permit the vulnerability by keeping connected to the deep well of truth and wisdom within as you watch the magic unfold.

We began, and so we will end, with intent, fully authentic spiritual intent; passionate intent; intent given in love, laughter and joyful playfulness, intent given from every aspect of your being, from your core. State that intention and commit to it. This type of commitment opens a door that can never close, gives knowledge you can never 'unknow,' sets into motion a wave of energy that cannot be halted, and sends an invitation to the universe. Intention is the first step through the door to the mastery of your destiny.

Chapter 7

LIVING THE MYSTERY

The seventh level for the ancient Egyptians was the great mystery. They entered the King's Chamber for three days and came out with the knowledge imprinted on their being.

You too have all the information you need within you.

You are not this physical body…

You are not your thoughts…

You are not your emotions…

You are not your past…

You are not your future….

You are more than you know you are

You are that voice in your heart

You are an amazing light being having a physical experience on this planet

A being that has taken millennia to evolve

A being capable of many things

Capable of living a fully realised existence on a fully conscious Earth

Living the 'present' you have been given – dreaming the Great Mystery.

One of the most colourful experiences I have ever had was during a meditation led by my Reiki master, Sue Richter. Sue guided the group back to Atlantis and told us to visit the temple. As I entered the temple courtyard, it seemed that the molecular structure of my whole energy being was morphing at a cellular level – continuously. I had the tangible sensation of shape shifting through all the possibilities of me, along with a knowing that I was absolutely splendid and powerful beyond all measure; it felt incredible.

Sue said I had "been in Lemuria." It meant little at the time, but later I got some clarity from Sekhem teachings around the idea that we all come into the world with a blueprint of perfection. For me, that clarity was about human potential, an idea that grew into 'You are more than you know you are', the basis of this writing. I got further confirmation that this had been a significant experience when I read Rudolf Steiner's account 'Egyptian Myths and Mysteries' of clairvoyantly viewing the potential of a rose and all the possibilities of that rose while it was in the birthing pool of its creation. His description was an exact reflection of how I had seen the possibilities of my potential self, and indeed, my past or future selves. Now, I don't know if there are parallel universes, altered dimensions, and past lives, or if my subconscious was giving me a colourful analogy. The science of it all has never interested me; the mystery and experience of it does. I certainly know there are many states of mind and a variety of realities. I encourage you to explore what that might mean for you.

Ah, so, the conclusion!

If you are not your body, your thoughts, your emotions, your past nor your future, then who are you?

As in all the mystery schools, the seventh step is the great mystery, the step you design yourself. The remainder is the voyage of discovery: the asking, watching, learning, living and loving.

You are more than you know you are.

The real you is already there, brimming over with potential and possibilities, and you are fully able to embrace the uncertainty and live in the mystery.

You are that voice in your heart.

It is the stillness within, the quiet secret of connection takes you beyond the illusion, beyond the pain, to wholeness and truth. As you look within, you'll continually surprise and delight yourself about who you actually are. The wisdom of the heart leads to an altogether gentler aspect of the self. Perspective taken from that place will throw a different light on situations and people. It will take you beyond the illusion of yourself, your ego self and your roles. We all get caught up in our small selves; it's easy to recognise. When you're fretting, iffing, butting or feeling irrationally hurt, it's a sure sign you're in ego. Ego keeps you asleep by being over-concerned with the mundane, but as you begin to see through the illusion of the self, you begin to see through the illusion of all things. Truly thinking for yourself, knowing yourself, mastering the small mind and connecting with the mind outwith the physical body, the universal mind, the collective unconscious, takes you deeper still. This mind field, or 'non-local field of information', which surrounds us in the same way that the magnetic field surrounds the Earth explains how we are able to connect with other minds, invisibly, the way one magnet is connected to every other on Earth.

"The field is indestructible. Fire cannot burn it, water cannot wet it, wind cannot dry it, and weapons cannot cleave it. It is ancient, it is unborn; it never dies." Deepak Chopra, Creating Affluence

You are an amazing light being having a physical experience on this wonderful planet

We've all experienced hunches, gut feelings, intuitive flashes, even sudden premonitions and other hints of foreknowledge. Who is on the phone before you pick up, or the presentiment associated with most great disasters...

...those who didn't go to work at the World Trade Centre on 9/11 because they felt suddenly sick or uneasy. Similar symptoms have kept passengers from flying on planes that later crashed. The French crew of the Concorde had dark premonitions before one of the supersonic jets crashed in 2000. Children felt uneasy going to school the day a coal-mine disaster engulfed a school in Wales in 1966, killing 144 people. One mother reported that her young daughter had a dream the night before of a black mass burying the school, which is exactly what occurred.

Imagine how that mother felt.

Listening to your instincts, hunches and dreams is another way of knowing yourself and tuning in to a deeper level of self-discovery.

Your Mind Is Outside Your Body

Mind outside the body could begin to explain some of those premonitions and why I have had a handful of incredible dreams that actually came true. Things I should not have known. Like what happened a long time ago when my daughter was just a toddler and we had the dog before Teddy, Fudge. A fellow seeker asked if I would accompany her to Findhorn. There she intended meditating with the divas to know which essences to add to a love potion she was creating, a new-age Red Bull, if you like. My home life didn't allow that kind of time out, so I apologetically declined, but agreed to tune in at the given moment. It came around just when Fudge was due his walk; that'd have to do.

I remember the day well. Sunny blue sky, hay baled for the first time that summer, a balmy stillness, precious and rare in Scotland. Far too glorious to sit inside in meditation. I remember that same friend had once told me about spinning; I'd never tried. So there and then, much to Fudge's confusion, I started turning around and around in the middle of the field. My spirit, already light from the energy of the day, soared with the sheer freedom of it. Soon I built up momentum and caught the rhythm I remembered feeling as a child. The essences just popped into my head without any effort at all.

I called my friend as soon as we reached home so that I could release my left thumb, which was clenched to remind me there were six. I'd gotten six out of the eight herbs she decided on. I knew then for sure that there was no need for fancy exercises to tune in to things we all already know. The spinning allowed me to shake ego to one side by simply being open, free and in nature, then the names of those herbs just popped into my head.

At first I was self-effacing about the whole thing, even put myself down for this 'skew-whiff' gift of mine that apparently emerged all the more, all the less I seemed to care. Then I realised I wasn't the only one. While teaching Sekhem, I made a cunning plan to encourage those who would say, "I can't feel the energy." Before beginning the exercise I'd do a drawing of where I sensed auric changes on the subject, then the student would 'guess'. I told them to pretend they did know, and they did know. It was amazing, and what self-confidence it gave. The funny thing was that those who overthought the situation were the self-proclaimed psychics! It made me laugh – dogma! You may as well throw it out with the cat litter.

Those were heady days during what seemed to be my bursary course direct from spirit, such experiences and lessons, but they're for another book, another day. For now I encourage you to find your own way of knowing, but whatever you find, trust it.

"The distinction between the past, present, and future is only a stubbornly persistent illusion." Albert Einstein

Research shows that premonition, or at least presentiment, is an everyday ability, at least to an extent. Dr Dean Radin, who worked on the Stargate programme, which studied psychic spying, became fascinated by the ability of 'lucky' soldiers to forecast the future and thus survive against the odds. Radin became convinced that thoughts and feelings, and occasionally, actual glimpses of the future, could flow backwards in time to guide them. So he hooked up volunteers to a modified lie detector and watched their reactions, - the electrical equivalent of a wince, to seeing either extremely violent, sexually explicit, or soothing images shown in random sequence. The volunteers began 'wincing' in the expected manner a few seconds before they actually saw the images! This experiment was repeated far beyond what chance alone would allow and is a great insight to the mind field's existence as an everyday affair.

Look at all of the examples of shared rhythms in nature: girls sharing a dorm end up menstruating at the same time and breastfeeding mothers will lactate when the baby cries even though their children are miles away. Also, any pet owner will tell you that their pet knows what they are thinking. In fact, researcher Rupert Sheldrake phoned up sixty-five vets in the London area and asked them if it was common for cat owners to cancel appointments because their cats had disappeared that day. Sixty-four vets responded that it was very common, and the sixty-fifth had given up making appointments for cats because too many couldn't be located when they were supposed to come in.

Sheldrake followed this up by putting dogs in outbuildings completely isolated from their owners, then asking the owner, at randomly selected times, to think about walking the dog for five minutes before going to fetch it. In the meantime, the dog was constantly videotaped in its isolated location. More than half the dogs ran to the door, wagging their tails, circling restlessly or otherwise showing anticipation of going for a walk, and they kept up this behaviour until their owners appeared, something none of the dogs did when their owners were not thinking about taking them for a walk.

"We're satisfied that people can sense the future before it happens."
-Professor Dick Bierman, psychologist at the University of Amsterdam

You Affect Everything Around You

Your 'antennae' are constantly bombarded with zillions of pieces of information. At the same time, you are emitting information to the universe. This has been proven over and over. In 1993, a group of scientists led by John Hagelin conducted an experiment in which several thousand people in Washington, D.C. meditated together twice a day for almost two months. This was correlated with highly significant reductions in crime.

"When two or more are gathered together in a common focus, the power to change the world is multiplied a thousand times more than if one person was doing it alone." Unknown

While the existence of this type of phenomena is clear, the reliability of it is less so. Nevertheless, at the very least these experiences prove there's still so much to learn.

You Are a Winner

Be the winner you are; you will be enacting the truth, because you are divinity incarnate, and your journey on this beautiful planet is your rite of passage. You earned it at the moment of your conception. It doesn't matter whether you believe that conception manifested due to the karmic contract you made with your soul group in order to learn the lessons for your soul's evolution; out of a biological certainty, when you won the race of life, one of three hundred million sperm; or as a gift from God/Goddess/All that Is. You made it, you are here, and are thus born a winner, born worthy. Worthy of this amazing life.

A being that has taken millennia to evolve.

You deserve an amazing life, for you are an amazing being. If you think about it, you truly are an amazing multi-dimensional creatures who has barely scratched the surface of all that you can do and be, yet you rarely stop to think just how incredible you truly are. Have a look at the BBC's Inside the Human Body and see the series of explosions fired off by the human egg at the exact moment of conception in order to prevent any other sperm entering. The big bang at the microcosmic level.

A being capable of many things.

The human body is the most complex creation in the universe. Your eyes can make over ten million colour distinctions; you can distinguish ten thousand smells. If your muscles all worked together in one direction, it would equal twenty-five tons of pulling power, all run by your incredible computer: the brain, which is housed in a body that will last over a hundred years with very little maintenance if properly cared for.

Wouldn't you love such a being? If you heard those facts in isolation, you'd be incredulous and perhaps think they were a description of an amazing spaceman, but that spaceman is YOU!

A spaceman that walks upright with feet that have 26 bones, 33 joints, 107 ligaments, 19 muscles and tendons, upon a rock, the third rock from the sun to be precise, that hurtles its way through space at an average velocity of 67,108 miles per hour and spins on itself at over a thousand miles per hour. Yet this rock is an amazing living, growing being just like you! She is your host and part of your purpose is to care for her. We named her EARTH, as that is where we physically connect with her: our soles to her earth. If you walk with your bare feet, especially in nature, in sacred places, you will connect even more – not only to her, but to the cosmos, to the whole of creation.

So, amazing being, spend your days in truth.

Spend today as a child of the cosmos.

The walls of the temples in Egypt depict a strong correlation between Earth and heaven, and the ancient Egyptians had total cosmic consciousness. They did not bother to differentiate between the sacred and the divine, so much so that what we now call religion did not even need a name. Heaven was Egypt. We should not differentiate either; we are both sacred and divine and this is heaven on Earth, right now!

"I like to walk alone on country paths, rice plants and wild grasses on both sides, putting each foot down on the earth in mindfulness, knowing that I walk on the wondrous earth. In such moments, existence is a miraculous and mysterious reality. People usually consider walking on water or in thin air a miracle. But I think the real miracle is not to walk either on water or in thin air, but to walk on earth. Every day we are engaged in a miracle which we don't even recognise: a blue sky, white

clouds, green leaves, the black curious eyes of a child – our own two eyes. All is a miracle." Zen Master Thich Nhat Hanh

Spend today as if your every act is a sacred symbolic gesture of the divine.

Continue to imagine going through your day as if you truly love yourself, feel worthy, whole and lovable. Knowing the truth of who you are, that each step on the road is your birthright and can be taken in love and in joy. One step after the other. You are amazing, divine, and worthy; keep reminding yourself and behave accordingly and you will attract the right people and experiences into your life.

Spend today as if you are truly worthy – gods and goddesses walking the Earth.

What is most amazing to me is that you are conscious; you have all these choices. You can set the default programme and continue to tweak it when events or circumstances require. You can choose your inner chemicals, your thoughts, and therefore, your emotions. You can put your desires and requests into the mystery, the quantum soup and again keep tweaking the ingredients until you find the recipe you desire, moment-to-moment, day-by-day.

Stay within and honour the present you have been given.

Take responsibility. You need to take responsibility for your needs so that you can grow, but there is little point if you do not take care of your body and of your home. So stop wasting and throwing away; buy stuff that will last, that you can reuse and repair. Buy products with toxin-free packaging, and prevent waste in the first place. Give to the charity shops, Freecycle, donate; don't use paper cups or napkins; reuse glass bottles and jars for leftovers; use refillable pens; use recycled and fair-trade products. You are not being all that you can be if you are not fulfilling your contract as caretaker of the planet.

Spend today as if you truly love your beautiful Earth, as if you truly love yourself.

Dreamer of the Great Mystery, I invite you to enter the Sekhem.

Glossary

Psychology
Psychology is the study of human behaviour. It seeks to understand the motivational forces within each individual, which explains his or her responses to the environment, especially to other people.

Psychotherapy
Psychotherapy is the application of psychological knowledge to the treatment of those suffering from disorders of a psychological origin.

Hypnosis
Hypnosis can be defined as a state of consciousness involving focused attention and reduced peripheral awareness and characterized by an enhanced capacity for response to suggestion. During hypnosis you will experience heightened focus and be able to concentrate intensely on a specific thought or memory, while blocking out sources of distraction.

Neuro Linguistic Programming
Although used by many therapists, Neuro Linguistic Programming or NLP, is not a therapy. Founder Dr Richard Bandler describes NLP as "an attitude and a methodology, which leaves behind a trail of techniques."

Neuro or the neurology relates to how we think and represent it to ourselves through our senses. Linguistic is about how we use language (verbal and non-verbal) to give meaning to our experiences and how that meaning affects us. Programming is how we turn those representations into behaviours and strategies to achieve our outcomes.

UKCP
The UK Council for Psychotherapy (UKCP) is the UK's leading professional body for the education, training and accreditation of psychotherapists and psychotherapeutic counsellors.

UKCP is the quality mark for high standards in psychotherapy. They hold the national register of psychotherapists and psychotherapeutic counsellors, listing those practitioner members who meet exacting standards and training requirements.

Yoga Nidra

The direct translation of Yoga Nidra is 'yogic sleep.' For absolute relaxation you must remain aware and awake, so we're talking about dynamic sleep, a systematic method of inducing complete physical, mental and emotional relaxation. During practice, your body sleeps, but you keep your senses of hearing and feeling alert, while lying still in absolute comfort. It is a beautiful experience which takes you into theta consciousness, a level of consciousness which lies between waking and sleep and within which, healing occurs.

When consciousness is separated from external awareness and sleep, it becomes very powerful and you can utilise it to develop memory, increase knowledge and creativity, even transform your very nature. Yoga Nidra can be used for directing the mind to accomplish anything. A powerful tool for achieving your goals, practicing Yoga Nidra gives you choice in life and that choice is created by the sankalpa.

Sankalpa

Sankalpa is a Sanskrit word which can be translated as 'resolve' or 'resolution.' You can think of it as a seed of intention, a powerful method of changing yourself and therefore the direction of your life from deep within. It is everything you've ever heard about affirmations with knobs on. We use it during the practice of Yoga Nidra.

There's a more detailed account in the Resources and Recordings for Mastering the Past.

Pranayama

'Prana' is breath or vital energy in the body. On subtle levels 'prana' represents the 'pranic energy' responsible for life or life force, and 'ayama' means control. So pranayama is 'control of breath.'

Sekhem
This is the explanation I was given as a trainee.

"Sekhem is a complete energy system and everything that is inherent and implied in that term. Sekhem works on a totally different concept and philosophy to other energy healing systems. And although there are some similar sounding systems, none can compare with this high vibrational energy that works at the very soul level. It assists you to take responsibility for your life, to heal, to grow both personally and spiritually and so become more of whom you really are.

Although you will hear that Sekhem is derived from the temples of very ancient Egypt it is even more ancient than that. It has come though Atlantis and Lemuria and has surfaced now to assist humanity change vibrational rate quickly and easily so that both mankind and the Earth may ascend to their higher purpose. As an individual it will take you back to your roots of power and then forward to the life you were always meant to live."

I wouldn't change a word.

Ancient Mystery Schools
During your journey you have learned the lessons of the ancient mystery schools: mastering the body, the mind, the emotions and the past; mastering destiny and living the great mystery which in every sense IS the life of your dreams. The mystery schools of ancient times were where a young apprentice or neophyte would enter to learn the secrets of the mysteries. The mystery schools of ancient Egypt have always epitomized the ultimate in secret wisdom and knowledge

Afterword

Thank you for reading the book, it has been a privilege sharing it with you, and I hope the beginning of a journey we will continue together.

In order to keep moving in the right direction I recommend noting what was most useful, what REALLY made a difference to you. Post it in your diary along with a reminder of what you need to do to look after and to love yourself - you deserve no less! I'd also love to know what the most helpful parts were. Knowing what did and didn't work, whether there was more I could have done, or anything I could have done differently, are key to my helping others in future, so your feedback is always appreciated. I love to read your testimonials too. What your experience was and what might help others. The best feedback of course is recommendations, that's how small businesses like mine grow - so do pass on my details.

Anyway now that you have read the book, it's time to begin going through the Resources and Recordings.

The main resource in all of this is of course is YOU!!! Your personal resources and discovering them, is the whole point! However when I refer to the Resources and Recordings I mean the resources that both explain and guide the 'how to' of The Me I Want To Be. It spells out how to sit for meditation, how to lie for deeper relaxations, how much water to drink, exactly how to talk to your subconscious mind and why these things work.

Over and above that I have recorded each and every meditation, relaxation and exercise, a total in excess of seven hours of audio downloads. Regular practice of these meditations will make them second nature, and before you know it you will be able to access these states at the drop of a hat. The relaxations and exercises are both cathartic and restorative. So once you have taken care of all the practicalities, like switching the phone to silent, you can really embrace them, trance is a natural state, so relax and enjoy it. My gift to you are these recordings, prepared with love so that you can trance out and enjoy them without doing a thing. Just settle down, get comfortable and listen to the sound of my voice. The whole work is known as **The Me I Want To Be: Resources and Recordings.**

As interesting as the book may be, the gold is in this part, the support behind it, the **how to be** *The Me I Want To Be*. I'd like to make sure you have it at your fingertips. So if you didn't get your downloads along with the purchase of your book you can pick them up now at: www.vickirebecca.com/resourcesandrecordings

Here's a little information about my one to one sessions, training and retreat work.

ONE TO ONE
As I am sure you already realise I believe that all of us can overcome anything that is standing in the way of the greatest and grandest expression of who we are. My one to one work is all about helping unlock that potential in YOU!

My style is informal, gentle, at times humorous, and at others quite direct and our session will be specific to your situation. Together we'll dramatically improve your mind set and overcome whatever is holding you back.

You can book me for one to one work on:
www.hypnotherapyaberdeen.co.uk
for either face to face or online sessions.

TRAINING
My purpose in the publication of this book has been to teach the core skills of personal growth including various means of relaxation and mind mastery. I do the same thing in classes and on retreats and coming soon, online webinars. The training consists of the things I feel really make a difference in helping people making the shifts they need to make.

In my time I have also trained hypnosis to diploma level, Sekhem to master level and Indian Head Massage to TLC level, and indeed still do in the right situation. My extensive background in health promotion, fitness training, yoga and meditation practice as well as professional qualifications to trainer level in advanced clinical hypnosis, NLP and psychotherapy has enabled me to take those skills to any level and still keep a holistic and very down to earth approach. I feel blessed by what that has brought me and delight in sharing it with lovely people like you.

RETREATS

This is my perk and who wouldn't want to be doing what they love in amazing places around the world! I have always had wanderlust, and over my years as a spiritual tourist have found that magical things happen when the right souls gather in incredible places. These days I team up with other professionals to share the places we love with our groups

During our retreats and tours we simply hold the space that allows you to step back and find that essence, that core, that purpose, and sit there for long enough to realign. We offer the type of training outlined above and other methods which will allow you to receive the messages you need to hear in order to walk fully into the greatest expression of your being.

To join us on one of our magical journeys go to www.spiritual-tours.co.uk

Here's a few other things you might also want to know.

To keep in touch you can receive my newsletter by signing up on:
www.vickirebecca.com/newsletter/

You may also want to join our little community on Facebook
https://www.facebook.com/groups/520822091399715/

Or pick up posts and events from my Facebook page
https://www.facebook.com/vicki.rebecca/?fref=ts

Any questions at all and you can message me on there or if you prefer email: enquiries@vickirebecca.com

The Me I Want To Be: Resources and Recordings can be picked up at: www.vickirebecca.com/resourcesandrecordings

Just about everything else can be found on www.vickirebecca.com

Printed in Great Britain
by Amazon

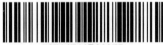